Inside The Priory

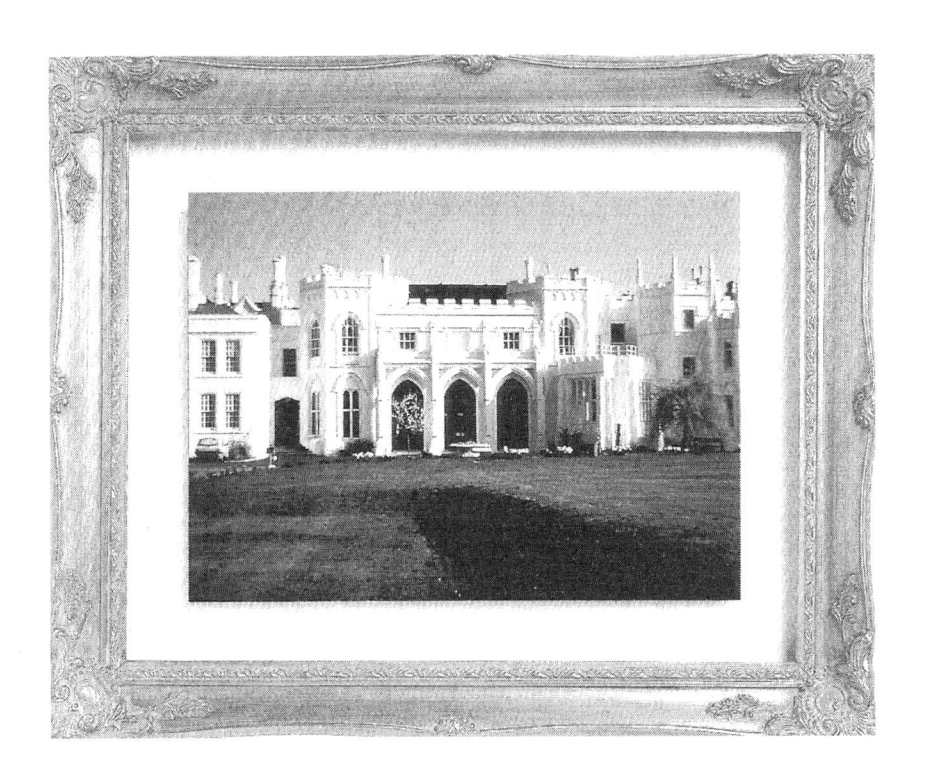

Dee Bixley

Copyright © Dee Bixley

The right of Dee Bixley to be identified as the author of this work has been asserted by her in accordance with the Copyright, Designs and Patents Act 1988.

A catalogue record for this book is available from the British Library.

ISBN: 978-0-7552-1495-2

All rights reserved. No part of this publication may be reproduced, stored in a retrieval system, or transmitted in any form or by any means, electronic, mechanical, photocopying, recording or otherwise, without the prior permission in writing of the copyright owner.

First Published in Great Britain 2012 by Bright Pen,
an imprint of Authors OnLine

Cover design © James Fitt

Also available as an eBook

For my son, Rob

CONTENTS

	Acknowledgements	*page*	vii
	Introduction		ix
1	My Voluntary Route Into Psychiatry		1
2	Going Private		5
3	An American Rocks Roehampton		11
4	The Nursing Persuasion		21
5	Trail Blazing Academy		33
6	Maintaining The Fabric		49
7	Dispensing Care		69
8	Naval Commander Opts For Dry Land		73
9	Gatekeepers of the Mind		87
10	Sleep Your Troubles Away		117
11	Last Chance Saloon		127
12	I Don't Want To See You Again!		153
13	Sanctuary		157
14	A Spiritual Slant		179
15	The Importance of Being Earnie		183
16	Princess Diana and The Priory		187

17 Going Public	193
18 Time Out	201
Sources	211
Seminars	213
Index	219

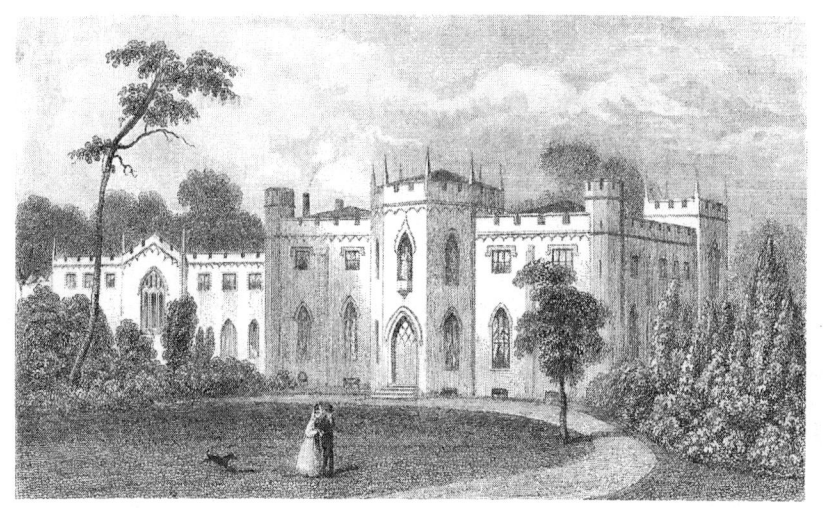

The Priory in about 1825, before the additions of Roumieu and Gough

A kind of abdication takes place when you pass through those glass doors. You feel like you are going into a sort of capsule of safety, where no one is going to turn a hair at your 'weird' beliefs – where people will see you and talk to you as someone who is suffering and not as someone who is bonkers. Therapy is great, medication is essential for some, but the alchemy of real healing lies elsewhere, and is intimately connected with such things as peace, kindness and the opportunity to breathe – all of which are available at The Priory.

a patient

Acknowledgements

My heartfelt thanks go to all the people within these pages who have helped to ensure that their fragments of The Priory's story are not forgotten. The record is the richer for their contribution.

Some have been particularly generous, such as Glorianna Murphy, who never complained when I phoned her at all hours to check out my facts; Brian Suter, who graciously lent me his front room to carry out some interviews; Jean Kilshaw, and the invaluable pages of Priory Hospitals Group (PHG) News. John Hughes, one-time Chairman & Chief Executive, who imparted humour and boosts to my morale in emails from all over the globe.

I would also like to thank medical historian Dr John Ford for his practical advice; author and raconteur Jeremy Thomas, who persuaded me to include my own story; Brian Pattinson, of the Book House in, Thame, Oxfordshire for his confidence in me, and Alex Fontaine MBE, who never ceases to delight and support me.

During my first week at The Priory it was my great fortune to meet a lady who became my 'surrogate Mum', Sheila Coyle. Sheila's positive influence on my life continues unabated, even though she has died. I will always be grateful for her love, enthusiasm, and constructive criticism.

Dr Desmond Kelly has been unstinting in his support and his wife Angela has welcomed me to their home and prepared scrumptious lunches, making book discussions even more pleasurable.

Most of all to my husband Mel, whose patience, humour and gentle persuasion has seen me complete this project. I don't think he has seriously thought about booking himself into The Priory as a consequence but I'm pretty sure he's thought of dropping me off there!

Front and Back Covers:

One of the 'Chelsea Artists', Ian Ribbons was originally asked to paint a watercolour of The Priory for a Christmas card (front cover). He spent three days on the lawn sketching, oblivious of the antics of patients around him. Later, he was commissioned by Dr Kelly to paint The Priory at night (back cover).

Introduction

Last night I dreamt I went to The Priory again; underneath the arches, through the glass doors to curling, creaky corridors. At first uncertain, I gained momentum as I sensed once more the security of those corridors, the way they seem to envelop and protect you. Weird and wonderful patients have stalked them for 140 years. They seemed never-ending in the dream and in reality that is what the road to recovery must feel like for Priory patients, a never-ending journey.

I worked at The Roehampton Priory, the famous private psychiatric hospital, for 15 years so you could say that this is an 'inside job'. My name was Dorothy White, and as Personal Assistant to the Medical Director, I found the experience so compelling that I vowed to capture someday the essence of the place. The stories in this book embody a span of time from the Fifties until the early 2000s. By then The Priory had changed hands (together with the other units that now form The Priory Group), entering yet another era in its intriguing history.

What better way to tell the tale than through the words of those who worked and were treated at The Priory? During a time of huge innovation in the treatment of addictions and behavioural disorders, staff and patients describe their own experiences.

I will be here to guide you along, introducing the chapters and writing about a few staff members and patients that I wasn't able to interview. I will also tell you some of my Priory anecdotes and about what was going on in my own life.

There can be no doubting The Priory's role in shaping the history of psychiatry: it is significant. Dr William Wood, who founded the hospital in 1872, couldn't possibly have predicted its transformation. From a little-known psychiatric nursing home it became a hospital admired for its academic excellence and accredited for training not only psychiatrists but general practitioners, medical students and nurses too. It achieved international recognition for its successful treatments and academic achievements. As an example, The Priory was voted Best Psychiatry Teaching Firm in 1997/98 by The Royal Free and University College Medical School students.

This metamorphosis began in the 1980s and doctors and staff explain how such unique academic recognition turned The Priory into a household name. Known as *the* place to have your nervous breakdown, celebrities flocked in and *The Official Sloane Ranger Handbook* described The Priory as '…a favourite Sloane bin where one's uncle goes to dry out'. What's more, it was gaining unique status as an independent teaching hospital.

Stigma and mental illness have always been associated. A lack of knowledge can make us mock behaviour we don't understand and this in turn can stop the sufferer from seeking help. As the Black Dog Tribe website created by Ruby Wax states - 'Mental illness does not discriminate, it does stigmatise.'

One boy's impression of what went on at The Priory, back in 1949, is summed up beautifully by James Morgan, who was at school nearby:

> "Nearly every day I would cycle to school from my home in Sheen. If one strayed further down Priory Lane there was always the mystery at the bottom. The Priory was hidden, hidden from view and hidden from comment. We children spoke of it in hushed tones; some would say it housed the mad relatives of the rich and royal, others that you would surely go mad, or be seized, if you ventured within that forbidding entrance. It was the only place in my cycling circuit where I never trespassed."

Before it became a hospital…

The Priory: it seems an unlikely name for a psychiatric hospital. In fact the building was a private home originally, built on land owned by Sir Thomas Bernard, 3rd Baronet, a wealthy barrister and treasurer of the Foundling Hospital. He purchased the land in 1800 and by 1811 The Priory must have been built because Sir Bernard sold for £11,000 '…all that capital messuage or mansion house at Roehampton… called The Priory'. It's possible that the name simply reflected the gothic romanticism of those times. The sale included 42 acres of land and the purchaser was Sir James Henry Craig (Governor of Canada, 1806-11).

By 1838 The Priory was owned by Sir James Lewis Knight Bruce, distinguished lawyer and judge, treasurer of Lincoln's Inn, and one of the first Lords Justice of Appeal.

Born plain James Knight in Barnstaple in 1791, he was called to the bar in 1817. Before he moved to Roehampton, he was noted for walking to Lincoln's Inn from his home in Ealing, a habit begun in earlier years when his health was so delicate he preferred to save the sixpenny coach fare to assist his family should he not return. He recalled how he would envy the gentry rattling past him in their carriages, but by 1835 his own income, at £18,000 was unequalled and he could afford to join them.

As a man of fortune and distinction, Knight Bruce felt that Bernard's creation should be improved upon to reflect his elevated status. So he enlisted the services of two architects noted for their gothic flamboyance, R L Roumieu and A D Gough. The pair worked in partnership between 1836 and 1848 and, turning their eccentric gaze on The Priory, they built a tower to the east of the original building, remodelled the main house, built an extension to the west and embellished the skyline with a forest of gables and elaborately carved chimneys. Their finished handiwork made Bernard's vision look almost austere and it delighted Knight Bruce who moved in with his wife, Eliza, and eleven servants around 1841.

Intriguingly, the journalist Rory Knight Bruce, who has written articles in the national papers about The Priory, is the great-great grandson of Sir James. A piece in the *Daily Express*, on 2 November 1996 - *'Detox deluxe'* - has the subtitle *'A hungover Rory Knight Bruce takes his liver back to the ancestral home, now a clinic, to dry out'*.

During his stay, Rory Knight Bruce witnessed many treatments and in summing up stated:

> "I left not resenting the old family home's new role. After all it has not fallen into decay, had a ring-road put through it or been turned into a hotel like Cliveden. Before my visit, all I had was an old print of my forebear. Now I have seen where he lived. "Do come again, any time," said Dr Desmond Kelly cheerfully as he showed me out to the Gothic porch. I considered asking for a family discount but felt too humbled."

...and when it became a hospital

The Priory's beginnings as a place of healing for the mentally sick started with Dr William Wood. As Resident Medical Officer at the Bethlem Royal Hospital (better known as 'Bedlam') between 1845 and 1852, Dr Wood was an enthusiastic pioneer of a more enlightened treatment of the insane, which transformed the old Bedlam into a modern hospital. He disliked the term lunatic and wanted the word asylum abolished. Of life as an in-house psychiatrist in a public asylum, Dr Wood later wrote:

> "There is, I suppose, no position in life where the nervous system is subjected to a more severe and continuous strain than that occupied by the medical superintendent of an asylum."

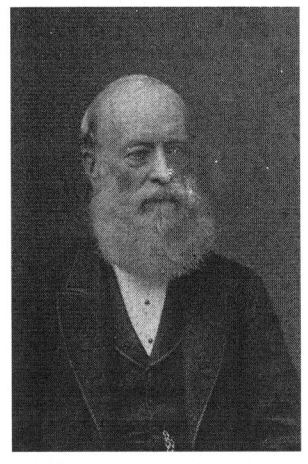

Dr William Wood

Eventually, Dr Wood joined the ranks of private asylum doctors when he took over Kensington House, a late seventeenth-century manor near Kensington Gardens. But when Kensington became less rural, he made enquiries and in 1870 he heard of a country house for sale at the tiny village of Roehampton in the County of Surrey. It was set in forty two acres of land with its own farm, and it was called The Priory.

Frankly, the property when he found it, covered in creeper, could not have enthralled Dr William Wood. Yet he saw its potential and its acreage and was particularly excited by the rookery in the elms on the front lawn. He invested large sums in alterations and extensions to the building.

So it was that on a damp June morning in 1872 an unusual procession made its way along the road to Roehampton, passing by fields and woodland until it reached a pair of carved oak gates guarded by a thatched lodge. Rattling along a driveway through parkland shaded by elms, oaks and beech trees, the carriages would have passed a field of cows and a farmyard and arrived at the main entrance to a manor house.

The forty-five people helped down from the convoy were dressed like gentry, the gentlemen in frock coats and neatly whiskered, and some of the ladies in new-fangled bustles. In the manner of gentry, they were attended by a team of maids in starched caps, as well as men-servants. But one or two of the gentlemen would probably have been without belts, braces or neckties, and firmly grasped by an attendant. Others might have been over-excited and gabbling to no one in particular.

The house looming over them looked impressive. It was a castellated building with grey stuccoed walls, the windows were gothic arches and frilly pinnacles rose black against the sky.

Dr Wood was a firm believer in the healing properties that architecture could have on patients' morale. He also knew the importance of first impressions:

> "The very aspect of the building to which the patient is often so unwillingly taken may make an impression on his mind most prejudicial to his recovery. It is not enough to provide for the animal wants and personal comforts... if the arrangement of the building itself suggests the thought of imprisonment."

Dr William Wood had hopes of creating at The Priory one of the finest private psychiatric hospitals in Britain.

And this is what it became.

1
My Voluntary Route Into Psychiatry

There are many ways to enter the world of psychiatry. My way was propelled by an over-zealous immigration officer at Kennedy Airport. It was September 1977. I had arrived at JFK from Heathrow minutes before and an officer didn't like the fact that I had no return ticket. My explanation, that I would be with my sister who had lived in America for many years, met with a stony stare. My length of stay, I continued, depended on how I liked the country. Despite the officer's assertion that I would be catching the next flight back to England, my sister came to the rescue with a lawyer and a $2,000 bond, to be returned if I kept out of trouble.

Hopefully (if I decided to stay) a Green Card allowing me to work would eventually follow and meanwhile, voluntary work would keep me busy. On my first day as a volunteer at St Raphael's Hospital, in New Haven, Connecticut, I was ready for anything. It was good to feel like a useful illegal immigrant.

The Chief Volunteer smiles warmly as she encourages me to "try passing some juices for me today, honey." It seems an odd request but this is America after all, and if a urine sample now means a Green Card later, so be it. She steers me towards a laden trolley and I realise that what she really wants me to do is hand out tubs of cranberry juice. I set off behind my supplies with a show of confidence.

The nurses are friendly on the wards: "Hi! How are you?" They don't really want to know. Those words seemed to invite thoughtful response when I first arrived in the States. But having been left mid-sentence a few times, my inquisitors long out of sight, I got smart. So now I march on with my wares, leaving a series of "Fine thanks!" in my wake.

My enthusiasm flags when confronted by patients in all manner of disrepair. The surgical wards in particular stimulate an ever-ready squeamishness. What's more, they don't all want my damned juice, "Get the hell outa here!" yells one guy, throwing the offensive liquid at my fleeing ankles.

One ward is off limits: Private One. A porter confides the reason: "It's the *Psych* unit," he whispers, stepping back to watch my reaction, which is instant fascination.

A few days later I manage to deliver mail to this mysterious place and Diane, the friendly secretary inside, just loves my accent. She's heavily pregnant and leaving soon. As we chat, I reach round to an itch on my back. It is an itch that will change my life because someone helps me scratch. I turn round to meet Gerald Flamm, Yale Professor and Chairman of Psychiatry. He too loves my accent and hearing of my secretarial background, ushers me to his inner sanctum with a brisk "Diane, hold my calls."

I have never met a psychiatrist before and hover nervously, worried that he'll analyse me. There is no sign of this as he seats himself comfortably, draws up a footstool and reaches for his pad. At last he's ready, an expectant pen poised. He looks just like Freud. "Tell me about yourself" he says. He speaks with inviting familiarity and in my mind's eye I see velvet cushions with *Trust Me* embroidered in silk.

I sit warily and babble. "I'm staying with my sister... she has lived in the States for years...I'm waiting for a Green Card...it's going to take months. So I'm a volunteer," I finish foolishly, in case he's overlooked my pink volunteer's jacket.

A few questions later, the professor reaches into the pocket of his white coat for a diary. "Joe Shulman's a good friend of mine, a Senator in Washington. He owes me a favour. Let's see if we can't get that work permit hurried up." Half an hour later I emerge with high hopes. Two weeks later I am initiated into the fascinating world of psychiatry.

All the psychiatrists on Private One seem glamorous and slightly wacky. They recognise an appreciative audience and regale me with stories packed with pathos. Dr Flamm seems a contented soul and when I remark upon this he says, "Don't know if I'm happy; don't stop long enough to find out."

At the end of my first Friday he bustles out of his office, "Right, get your coat – TGIF", and happy hour cocktails on Friday become a ritual when he's in town.

Dr Flamm chairs various psychiatric associations, which means he's often away. During these quiet times I become friendly with the hospital's medical photographer. Her name is Doris but I'm to call her Huck, I don't know why. Her type of photography doesn't bring her to Private One, she says, but would I be interested in joining her one afternoon as she does her rounds? "Yes please" I gush, without the slightest idea what this entails.

By the time we reach the morgue and the sights and smells therein, I believe Huck senses my limitations. I can't enter the room, preferring to cling to the doorframe. On balance (and it's a grim choice) I prefer accompanying her to the wards, where she photographs cancerous livers and enlarged hearts, on slabs of green. This is the only time I go with Huck on her rounds.

Dr Flamm's patients include some ladies whose problems do seem rather minor and there is one in particular that he has trouble staying awake for. When she comes out to my office and throws herself on the spare chair with a forlorn "Asleep again," I'm dismayed and amused in equal measure. I listen to her problems until the doctor emerges cheerily. "Ah! Thought I'd find you here. Where were we?"

It emerges that most of my colleagues on Private One are undergoing Freudian analysis. It is an alien concept to me but since they all do it there must be benefits. When I quiz Dr Flamm about it he advises that I should have analysis myself. I'm extremely dubious but he is persuasive: "I have contacts," he insists. "It will be a fraction of the usual cost! It will only be 50-minute sessions five days a week for about four years."

By the time this stark reality hits home, and I attempt to sidestep the waiting couch, it is too late. I am committed to a process of vetting and before I know it I have my own lady analyst. During our initial face to face meetings, when we're assessing if we want to work together, I realise that she is all I want to be - studious, stylish, low-voiced and enigmatic.

At first, lying on a couch for 50 minutes during my lunch break, uttering whatever enters my head to the silent presence behind me (who could well be asleep) gives me alarmingly erotic dreams. These get narrated too and before long my ramblings deepen. I begin to look forward to my daily unburdening.

But after six months and with another Connecticut winter looming, I'm getting restless. California sounds particularly appealing. My analyst is perplexed and irritated. "Stopping now," she warns, "will be to give up something of great future value. You will be stuck in the mud of old patterns." I decide to take the risk.

I try to explain myself to Dr Flamm but he's disappointed in me too. He had thought that a nice long analysis would be just the thing to keep me happily working for him. But we write to each other and when he visits San Francisco for a psychiatric convention (together with a whole bunch of other shrinks from Connecticut) I'm invited to dine with them all.

After a year in San Francisco, and with my mother ill in hospital, I return to England. An advertisement in the crème de la crème section of *The Times*, for a personal assistant to the medical director of a private psychiatric hospital, sounds promising. They're looking for someone with 'superior initiative and superior skills'. I apply anyway and that's how I end up on leafy Priory Lane.

Let's start with the story of my erstwhile boss.

2
Going Private: why I left the NHS

Dr Desmond Kelly
Priory Years:
Medical Director (1980 - 1997)
Chairman, Priory Hospitals Group (1988 - 1993)
Chairman Emeritus & Group Medical Director (1993 - 1999)

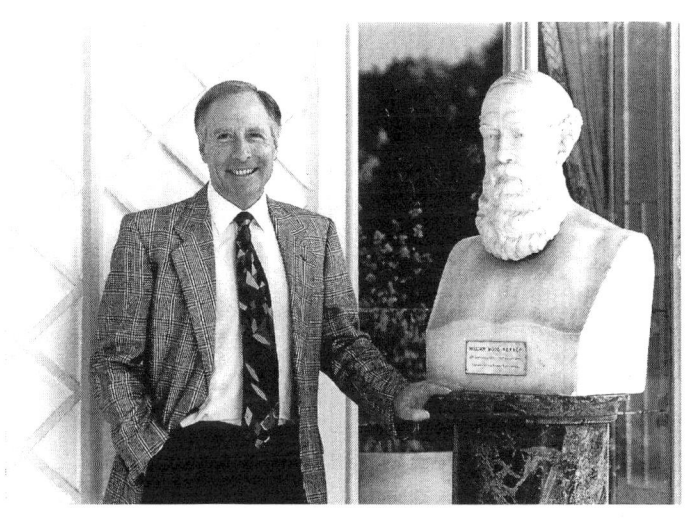

Dr Kelly with a bust of Dr William Wood

When he retired in 1999, Dr Kelly became Honorary President, Priory Healthcare. Phew!

"By the late Seventies, I had worked at St George's Hospital in London for ten years, mainly at its branch at Atkinson Morley's Hospital (AMH) in Wimbledon, where the inpatient departments of neurosurgery, neurology and psychiatry were based. I was a 'maximum part-time consultant', which enabled me to do a small amount of private work, and I was wondering about the next phase of my career.

I enjoyed treating patients in the NHS and privately. The only difference was that there was more time given to the private patients; this was what they were paying for.

I had been admitting my private patients to The Priory, and on occasion I was invited by John Flood, the Medical Director, and the other Priory consultants, to see patients for a second opinion.

It has to be said that when I first visited the Priory Nursing Home (as it was then called) it reminded me of Dracula's castle. I drove up a pitted drive through an avenue of trees to a building covered in ivy; I half expected bats to swoop out of the castellated turrets. A statue of a Prior, presiding over the front door, was the finishing touch. In fact, the Prior is now over the back entrance, because when a large piece of The Priory's land was sold to the Greater London Council in the late Sixties, the back became the front. So now the visitor sees that magnificent Strawberry Hill Gothic building in silhouette against the London sky. And no ivy.

The Priory had asked me to leave the NHS and join the hospital as a full time consultant. I thought about it for a long time but turned it down. To leave a London teaching hospital in the late 1970s to join an independent hospital that had been bankrupt 10 years before seemed a risk too far. But when they asked again in 1979, I accepted. With one condition: that I would become Medical Director in February 1980, when John Flood was due to retire. Knowing how risky the independent sector was, if the ship went down I wanted to be at the helm. Friends at St George's thought I was completely off my trolley!

Quite apart from abandoning the safety of the NHS, it was difficult to imagine leaving it for emotional reasons. I had been there man and boy during its golden era, when patients rarely complained about the service they received, knowing they were on to a good thing compared with the health system pre and post-war.

By the time I left St George's there had been a strike amongst the union staff, who wanted a closed shop. Many of the consultants became strike breakers and worked in the laundry and other departments to keep the hospital running. It was an ugly time in the NHS yet my loyalties were torn. I felt guilty about leaving my patients behind (even though I would be replaced by a very good consultant) and I was determined to continue seeing a few of my old patients without charge.

Most of all, I wanted to leave behind the myriad committees. Like other consultants, I turned up to defend my particular specialisation; surgeons and physicians were fighting for space, research funds and other commodities linked to the NHS.

I had of course felt responsible for inpatients on the psychiatric floor of AMH. It was an extremely difficult ward to defend against suicides, with open staircases that patients could jump off. Worst of all was the roof, with a grid of fire escapes around the building that patients could get to.

My worst moment there was when a patient got on the roof. A student nurse went up to talk him down, of her own volition. It wouldn't have taken much for them both to go crashing to their deaths. She was a very brave lady who produced a happy ending.

The responsibility at The Priory would be huge, especially the ability to influence events, and I was acutely aware that other people's jobs would depend on me. Still, you can leave a challenge until you are too old.

One of the first things I did as Medical Director was to change the name to The Priory Hospital. There is a world of difference between a nursing home and a hospital. Previously, The Priory had a large number of long stay patients, many of whom brought in their own furniture. But 'acute' psychiatry aims at getting people better in the shortest possible time and major advances in treatment now made this possible.

We began a series of seminars, inviting general practitioners, psychiatrists and therapists to attend. The chef's delicious lunches were the perfect prelude to afternoons of clinical and academic excellence, and these seminars were an essential factor in the changing culture of the place.

I realised that to make The Priory viable in an increasingly competitive market was going to be very stressful. Fortunately, stress was an area of research I'd been interested in, especially stress in the medical profession. I did not want to repent in intensive care following a coronary or some other awful event. A sick doctor can't help anyone.

I chose Transcendental Meditation (TM), which requires 20 minutes morning and evening. The morning proved easy. For me, meditation produced more benefit than sleep minute for minute, so it was simple to get up twenty minutes earlier.

Originally, when I got home from The Priory, my mind racing, I would have a glass of wine – after saying hello to my spaniel and wife in that order! When I started to meditate a lot of ideas would go through my mind at the same time as the mantra. After 20 minutes I would be much more relaxed and at peace with myself after the stress and strain of a Priory day. I got much more from it than a glass of wine. It seemed to quiet my overloaded brain and good ideas would appear. Many of my worries had been turned off.

I continued with this routine until I retired in 1999. It's so simple: sit on a chair (you don't have to be cross-legged on the floor), shut your eyes and recall a mantra [a particular sound with no meaning, therefore no tendency to distract you].

Transcendental Meditation reached millions worldwide but the Maharishi's aspirations were massive: 'If TM were performed by just 1% of the population' he insisted, 'the flow of good vibrations would flood over the nations of the world and bring about a universal state of bliss consciousness.'

My own ambitions were relatively modest: to make The Priory the best psychiatric hospital in the country."

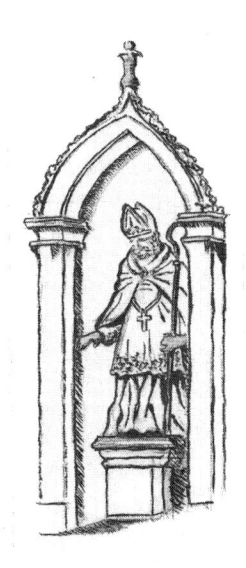

The Prior

***

My own connection with The Priory started when I responded to the advertisement in *The Times* and my interview was just before Christmas 1981. It was snowing as I walked the two miles from Putney Station. Rounding the corner of the drive and seeing that glorious building surrounded by fresh snow I thought: *what a place to work!* I gazed in awe as I surreptitiously pulled off my snowy boots for more elegant footwear and picked my way to the door. Strange to relate, it felt like coming home.

Dr Kelly seemed a very nice chap. By now I was used to psychiatrists, although he wasn't your obvious shrink. Dr Flamm in the States had been a typecast Freudian figure but Dr Kelly seemed more like a diplomat. After the interview he gave me a tour of the hospital, carried out at breakneck speed.

Christmas trees adorned the wards and nurses greeted the doctor cheerfully. Hastening after him I began to want the job desperately; to have a role in this swish and quirky place. Then two other psychiatrists interviewed me – possibly for second and third opinions as to my sanity. The present incumbent of the job interviewed me too - she was leaving with her husband for a post in Singapore. The ladies in the Secretariat (I would be their head of department) were quite a bit older than me and rather Sloane Ranger types. That was the Friday. On the Monday, they called to say the job was mine. I was ecstatic.

One task during my first week was to despatch a couple of hookers. They had been smuggled in by a recently admitted Arab but discovered in his room before any unseemliness could ensue. I was instructed to get rid of them pronto and snatched up the nearest phone to call a cab, "Er, where would you like to go?" I enquired.

The ladies debated and intriguingly the place that came out tops was Marble Arch. This was going to be a fascinating job.

I quickly learned that Dr Kelly (or 'DK' as I called him) had a special interest in patients with obsessive traits. There was a good reason for this; he had his own little checking rituals (annoyingly justified occasionally) and was a compulsive list maker. And he liked to get several of us doing the same thing... just to make sure. We would bump into each other attempting the same task – there would be a kind of Kelly conga of us – all charging to do what had already been done by the one in front. "Assumption" he would intone, "is the mother of cock up."

I could be obsessional too but DK's areas of obsession seemed unnecessary to me. This was exceedingly unfair, however, because for someone with dyslexia, he was remarkable. To have survived medical school and all those exams with dyslexia, and then to have climbed to the top of his tree seemed pretty amazing to me. No wonder he checked and re-checked everything.

Dr Kelly's patients meant a lot to him and they sensed this. His capacity for getting people to do what they didn't want to do was legendary but he found it difficult to say no to their demands sometimes. So I had to say it for him, causing one patient to complain: "She guards you like a lioness!" Others were more understanding – "...well, don't bother him. He's got so many nuts on his tree."

DK's reputation attracted patients from all over the world. I remember an American lady who crossed the Atlantic for the treatment of her paranoid delusions – she believed the world to be a very dangerous place. It was her first day in England and she was having her initial appointment with DK in the tranquillity of his office. I was working nearby and suddenly heard what sounded like a gunshot. In a madcap attempt to protect my boss, I did the unthinkable and barged in on a psychiatric consultation. I found him unhurt, unfazed and inspecting a hole in his window. As to the American lady, she looked vindicated, as if to say, you see? The world *is* a very dangerous place. The police said later that it was the prank of a kid with an air gun. My subsequent remonstrations that Dr Kelly should not sit in full view of the window were (quite rightly) ignored.

It was within my first week at The Priory that I had a stark demonstration of just how sick patients can be. It was dark as I walked out, musing over the day, when suddenly a woman pelted past me and out into Priory Lane. I instinctively dashed after her but it was too late: she had been run over and was lying in the road. This, of course, had been her intention. Nurses quickly appeared and I got out of the way. I felt shaken and terribly sorry for the woman and for the driver and for everyone else concerned. Guilty, too, that I hadn't been able to do anything. I was phoned later and told that she would recover.

Inside The Priory

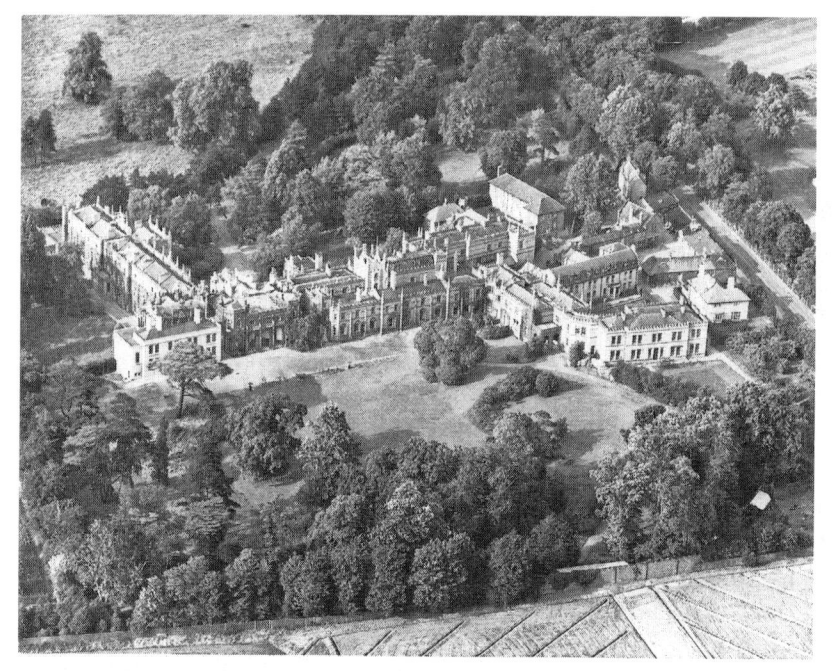

Aerial View of The Priory, 1961

3
An American Rocks Roehampton

John Hughes, Chairman & Chief Executive
Priory Years: 1980 – 1987

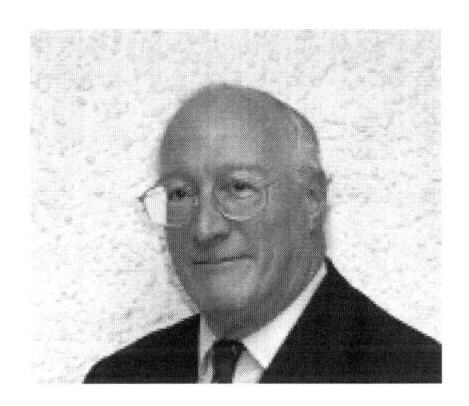

In 1980 John Hughes acquired The Priory on behalf of the American company Community Psychiatric Centers (CPC) and he built the first seven Priory hospitals. He went on to become Founder and Chief Executive of Cygnet Health Care, with 16 UK psychiatric hospitals and nursing homes.

John, who has described himself as a 'psychiatric hospital junkie', was awarded the Laing & Buisson Outstanding Contribution to Independent Healthcare Award in 2008. He has played a major role in shaping independent health provision in the UK.

"In 1979 the Thatcher government came into power and immediately released exchange controls, permitting the free movement of capital in and out of Britain for the first time since 1939. This set off an explosion of domestic as well as overseas capital investment in Britain and British outward investment abroad. The CPC purchase of The Priory was a tiny part of this phenomenon.

CPC, founded in 1968 was, by 1980, one of perhaps 20 hospital management companies listed on the New York Stock Exchange. The American version of 'privatisation' had increased these companies' market share from about 2% in 1970 to 5% in 1980, at the expense of mainly state-owned hospitals. CPC and others were acquisitive and expansion-minded.

Leading up to the acquisition of The Priory, in early 1980 I came over on behalf of CPC to scout the town and I looked at The Priory and Bowden House Clinic, and did a bit of industrial espionage for a week, looking at various units.

At the same time, Charter [Charter Medical, another big American hospital chain, which arrived in London the same year] also looked at The Priory. But they took the step of buying a unit and developing a clinic in Chelsea, and starting from scratch because they reckoned that they had the world's best answer to bringing modern psychiatric services to this quaint little country.

We looked at it quite the other way around, which was that it was much better to take what we found of the establishment, the structure of a hospital, and try to improve the bits that needed improving and build on the bits that worked pretty well. So my recommendation to the company was that they go for the acquisition of The Priory.

I gleaned an overview from my investigation, which was reinforced many times after the purchase was completed. The public view of private psychiatric hospitals in general and of The Priory specifically was that they were small, decadent places, sheltering a hotchpotch of wealthy, addled old ladies and alcoholic gentlemen of all ages. The triumphant Envy of the World, the National Health Service, ignored these places during the nationalisation wave of 1948-50. They declined the opportunity to acquire them for free. For five years or more after the 1980 acquisition, if I got into a taxi and said 'The Priory in Roehampton, please', the driver would often look round at me to size up the risk of my urinating in his cab.

The Medical Director, John Flood, was very unwell and it was realised that it wasn't necessarily a long term situation and they decided in 1980 to sell the place. We acquired both The Priory and Galsworthy House, which at that time was a free-standing unit on Kingston Hill, purchased by The Priory in 1978, and set up as a 12-step alcoholism treatment centre. The purchase price at completion in September 1980 was £2.2 million, of which £2.0 million was for The Priory and £0.2 million for Galsworthy House. We thought that was a fairly full price. At the time, the combined units were losing about £100,000 a year. It took me about three months after the acquisition to appreciate that roughly that amount was being stolen from the hospital every year and it took another three or four months to set that right by making a few changes of personnel. That probably doesn't bear too much description.

One very sad thing is that prior to our acquisition of the place, in something like June 1980, when we were first getting involved in serious discussions, Dr. Flood was stabbed by an intruder in his house, Priory Lodge. I think the stabbing was not in itself terribly serious and the intruder ran off, but Dr Flood died on the 4th July 1980. I remember the date quite specifically, not just because it was American Independence Day but because that was the day my plane landed at Heathrow, to finalise negotiations and purchase the place. I arrived to find out that Dr. Flood had died earlier that day.

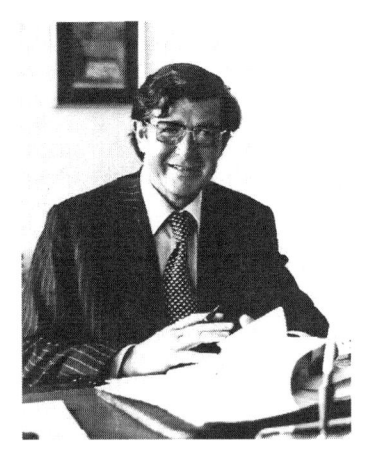

Dr John Flood

A few days later we had Dr. Flood's funeral, which was one of my most freeze frame déjà-vu moments. It was like stepping out of a full Technicolor movie into black and white. I asked whether it was appropriate – should I attend the funeral? And of course they said 'Oh yes, please do.' So I attended, for the first and perhaps last time in my life, the funeral of someone I had never met.

The funeral was like a Felliniesque parade of strangers, planted in a black and white dreamland - a big parade of hundreds of people. There I was, not quite belonging. I suspect that a few of the old time staff and people of simpler persuasion were somewhat superstitious. Some thought there was an omen in the fact that this fellow with the strange American accent and the foreign moneybags had arrived on the same day that Dr. Flood died.

There was a receptionist by the name of Bridie Gready who I never met. Bridie was an unmarried lady who was on reception at The Priory for many years. In fact when we took the place on in 1980 it still had one of those telephones you see in the movies with the lady with the earphones and the cords that you punch into slots in the switchboard. So that was what Miss Gready did all of her career. When they ran out of money in 1970, apparently Miss Gready loaned The Priory £5,000 of her life savings. This was a very substantial sum for somebody who was probably on £500 a year. I recall that as part of our completion arrangements we agreed to continue honouring an ex-gratia annuity of £200 per year. This sort of anomaly was unknown in America, so it seemed very odd to me.

The Board Room, even in 1980, was a quintessentially old-fashioned place. The doctors and the two or three most senior managers went into the room for a weekly lunch. In those days you would get a little thimble glass full of sherry and you would hold it just so and sip your sherry before they served you lunch.

Of course not much business would be discussed because it really wasn't quite the British thing to do. That would take place afterwards.

One of my first impressions was the contrast between the elegance of the Board Room, which was nicely decorated, had a glorious chandelier, very valuable antique furniture and a lovely board table, compared with the overall shabbiness and tackiness that the patients and particularly staff had to work with in the rest of the hospital.

The first encounter was for a welcoming lunch. Beforehand, everyone assembled at the big bay window at the front and we had our glasses of sherry. Looking out at the reserved spaces in the car park, they were all discussing the relative merits of Rolls Royce vs. Mercedes vs. Jaguar. My reactions to this were two – first: 'these people are whistling while Rome burns' - the place was losing money like a leaking hand basket and they were thinking about the status of one another's cars. Secondly, they were completely ignoring the fundamentals of how do we both improve patient care, and get more patients into this old turkey? I thought *what the hell am I going to do with this place? Do we really want to buy this or is Charter right: we should start from scratch?*

The negotiations got extremely protracted. I was then 33 years of age, and had developed a dozen or so hospitals in the United States in different regions. I had seen some fairly eccentric and regional differences in the States. But I was not at all prepared for the art of a British strategic delay in spinning out negotiations - driving the adversary quite mad through throwing in little irrelevancies and little delays. The art of strategic delay is to get just to the point when you hope the other guy caves in and signs, before he walks out instead.

It's a British game; I've learned how to master that now. You can turn it the other way round and drive the British adversaries stark raving mad by just letting things sit and not replying to letters and so forth. Initially it made me very angry. It took me about 12 months to overcome my instinctive American response, which was to pound my fist on the table and say 'I want it by Tuesday or I'm going to my lawyer!'

Dr. Flood, who was a good Irish Roman Catholic, had a number of priest and nun patients, referred by the Church. Initially there were three or four nuns in full habit circulating about the place. In our negotiations the people I was dealing with kept referring to the term 'nursing sister' – Sister Renée, Sister Eileen and so on. I assumed, from American English usage (a nurse is a nurse, never a sister), that they were referring to these nuns. I kept asking for copies of all the sisters' contracts of employment. I was told time after time that I had been given all of the sisters' contracts to review. I lost my patience:

'No! Surely there must be some sort of master contract which says where you're getting these damned nuns from. I haven't seen anything to the effect that you're paying the Cardinal or the Archbishop or the Mother Superior a penny for their labour.' They all fell about laughing because it seemed that we had one particularly long-staying nun as a patient and the other three were simply regular visitors!

The place was down at heel and in poor decorative state, in spite of the fact that there were 11 maintenance men. There were lovely old overstuffed chairs with springs sticking out in your rear end, and the fabrics worn off. There were parts of the roof in North Wing, where you could look up through the holes in the plaster of the ceiling and literally see sky and have pigeon droppings hitting patients' pillows down below.

Within a month of doing the deal and moving in and managing the place, I was unsettled by how calm things were. It just didn't seem normal to me. I hadn't seen a patient throw a plate or have a wild outburst. That was the sort of thing I was used to in America. It struck me as unusual. The patients were more or less the same, also the nature of their illnesses, and the medications we treated them with.

Yet the place had a much calmer aspect. Despite the general shabbiness, all patients had a private room. This was rare then in both America and Britain. I became thoroughly convinced that it's all down to privacy and physical environment for the patients. Therefore, in some ways we went over the top when renovating to make new units very comfortable and decoratively attractive. There may be cultural differences, in that Americans are noisier and more demanding generally. Perhaps they make a little more noise when they're mentally ill. I'm convinced that a large part of the relative calmness is down to having single rooms, with their importance in restoring normal sleep patterns and enhancing self-respect.

We inherited in September 1980 a patient occupancy of about 20 acute patients and about 50 psychogeriatric patients. Of the 20 acute patients, perhaps half of those were Arabs and the other half were British. All the long stay patients were British. I made the decision very early on to freeze the occupancy on the geriatric wards and we ran that down by attrition – as these old folks passed away, we didn't replace them.

The decision to change to more acute patients was very worrisome to the staff but not to the doctors. They understood the principles quite well and also wished to modernise the hospital. But the staff looked at the geriatric patients as the bread and butter of the place. The fact of the matter was that we were losing money on that end of the business.

Some patients were paying as little as 14 guineas a month (£14.70), on 'lifetime' contracts, from old trust funds that had been established before the days of galloping inflation. It was unsatisfactory, but of course we honoured the contracts. It was also clinically not the right thing to mix the psychogeriatric patients with the acute patients, who had much more positive prognoses. If you're 30-something and suffering from a depressive breakdown, you don't want to share your lunch with Major 'H' who's 96, badly socialised, and not a good role model.

The 'Narcosis' Ward was where the most difficult patients would go, where Dr.

Sargant used to do narcosis therapy. He would put patients to sleep for a week, two weeks at a time. They would be roused occasionally to get chicken soup but essentially they would sleep through their psychoses. Narcosis was done principally before the days of the modern anti-psychotic medications.

In the early Eighties we used to get a considerable number of patients from quite primitive backgrounds in Middle Eastern countries. We'd have ordinary foot soldiers and policemen and people who literally rode camels in their daily work in Saudi Arabia and Kuwait. Some of these men had never seen running water and this led to a combination of problems. You have a fellow suffering an acute psychosis at the same time that you are trying to toilet train him, and he was being nursed by a woman who was walking around without a veil. Women of that kind were seen as prostitutes to many of these guys.

Sister Eileen, who was in charge of the Narcosis Ward, described very eloquently how they handled one particular patient. I said, 'How is Mr. Al so-and-so getting along?' and she said 'Oh we put him in the bath.' Before that particular wing was remodelled they had this great Victorian claw-footed metal bathtub that would hold about six people if you wanted to have a party. It certainly held Mr. Al so-and-so very comfortably. The nurses filled it up with water and explained that the doctor had ordered that he must have a medicinal bath. He had to take his clothes off and get in the bath. He would be there for exactly one hour. They put a clock up as part of the ritual. Then they very carefully measured out cups of different coloured shampoos and other concoctions into the bathtub to calm this chap into sitting and taking his medicine for an hour. He came out much cleaner than when he went in.

There were some wonderful personalities amongst the staff. Doris Day, the tea lady who had worked there since 1953, told a story about the day Dr. Flood unlocked the doors of The Priory. When he became Medical Director in 1956 (and perhaps for a year after that), virtually all the wards and many private rooms were locked, with the original Victorian clanking keys.

Doris remembered as a youngster sliding patients' meals through slots underneath the doors in the locked units. Patients would stay there locked up for many years. Suddenly one day - it seemed like a lightning bolt to the staff – Dr. Flood gave the order that all the doors were to be unlocked. It seemed to many as though a ten megaton explosion had been ordered but nothing happened! It was perfectly all right and there was no reason for the doors to be locked. That gives you a glimpse of what was, even in 1958 or so, a very old-fashioned place. They were probably under some pressure at the time to comply with the (then current) Mental Health Act.

The *lingua franca* in the kitchen was Italian. One cook, Tony, had quite a thick accent. He had a pet pigeon that hung out on a freezer that sat in a semi-outdoor enclosure at the back of the kitchen. Needless to say it was a filthy, unsanitary situation, with a pigeon living there. I directed the department head to make Tony get rid of this pigeon one way or the other. So he took it away.

But it kept coming back. We had a chat with Tony when the pigeon came back the second time. In his broken English he said: 'I've a-taken-a-the-pigeon-a three times to Clapham-a-Junction-a-train station. I leave him there but he fly in the air and comes-a back-a.'

In the whole profession of psychiatry now there are few of the old breed of workaholic doctors. I wouldn't say they're all nine-to-fivers but most lack the pace and zeal of people like Desmond Kelly and David Thompson, his one-time Deputy. David, when I first met him, used to take the stairs up to the offices three at a time, in his rush and enthusiasm to get to the patients. I think probably by the time I departed he was down to taking them two at a time.

Desmond was extremely helpful through those years. I can't think of a single disagreement we had of any fundamental nature. He coins wonderful one-liners, and there was one that hit it on the head as an oblique compliment: 'Yes', he said, standing up to introduce a seminar, 'Here at The Priory we combine the best of British medicine with the best of American management.' He did not elaborate on any comparison with British management or American doctors!"

> See more from John in the chapters *Sleep Your Troubles Away*, *Last Chance Saloon*, and *Maintaining The Fabric*.

When a GP made a referral to Dr Kelly my first step was to contact the patient and set up an appointment. The Priory attracts many well-known people so it isn't unusual to recognise the name of the patient. But on one occasion it was the address I recognised. I had actually worked at that address in Berkshire as an *au pair*, for a family who eventually moved abroad.

As it happened, the Berkshire patient only needed to see the doctor a couple of times but months later, during an emotional trip back to the area, I found myself walking up the patient's drive and ringing his doorbell. (I never admitted this to DK). The ex-patient opened the door and I re-introduced myself. Outwardly, he showed no surprise at seeing me and calmly led the way through to the living room to meet his wife. But inwardly the poor man must have been thinking, what the heck is going on? I see a shrink a couple of times and months later his secretary turns up on my doorstep? (No wonder I never told DK).

He and his wife listened to my story. You see, I had a son, Robert Jamie, in 1970 and he had been adopted from this very address in 1972. I was asking them to let me know if he ever came looking for me. I knew the chances were miniscule but I had to cover all possibilities.

One of my last memories of Robert was in that living room, when he toddled over to where I was sitting on the floor drying my hair. At full and important height, he stretched his arms out for a long and trusting snuggle while the drone and warmth of the hairdryer mesmerised us both. By then, I had made the decision that would part us. But my little boy didn't know that soon he would go to live with a mythical couple who had everything: everything but him.

It is no exaggeration to say that I thought of Robert every day in the years that followed his adoption. I clung to the belief that if he had anything like my curiosity (and no matter how happy he was with his adoptive parents), some day he'd come looking for me.

In an attempt to help this along, in September 1987 (five years after I began working at The Priory) I tracked down the adoption society. They had moved from WC1 to SW4 and having summoned the courage to phone them, it was heartening to learn that their records went back 70 years, so they would certainly have our file. They seemed really pleased to hear from me and I got the impression that not many 'birth mothers' initiated contact. I followed up with a letter, asking them to keep it on file in case my son got in touch.

Acknowledging my letter in October, they wrote:

> "…It was lovely to hear from you again after all this time and we will certainly make a note on your file as you request. If, therefore, your son Robert makes enquiries about you and wishes to contact you we will, of course, let him know you have been in touch with the Society. Robert himself so far has not exercised his right under Section 26 of the Children Act 1975 and as you know he must start the ball rolling. The Act conferred no new rights on natural parents. There is nothing more you can do at this stage

but rest assured that we have your name and address. If you move, it would be as well to inform us."

A previous letter from the society had been dated 2nd October 1972:

"…At a recent Court Hearing the Adoption Order was granted for baby Robert. Please be assured he is very happily settled with this family and greatly loved and they hope to have a sister for him when he is a few months older. We shall not be writing again, so would like to wish you much happiness in the future."

4
The Nursing Persuasion

Unfortunately, I missed the opportunity to interview Betty Naudeer, who was the Director of Nursing at The Priory from 1982-1994. Her title encompassed the traditional role of Matron.

Betty greeted new patients, saw them all each day, and remembered everyone by name. I loved it when she included me on her rounds, popping in to see how the world was treating me.

Betty had previously worked at Queen Mary's Hospital, Roehampton, and her appointment at The Priory (her first venture into the private sector) strengthened the links between the two hospitals. From the start, she was enthusiastic about The Priory but knew she had to make changes; psychiatry was changing and so was the political situation.

Mrs Naudeer ensured that the number of nurses on the wards related to the severity of illness and intensity of nursing care required, rather than to the number of patients. There were 80 nurses, and a 'nurse bank' of 65 staff provided cover for illness and holidays. This meant a nurse/patient ratio of one to four, which Mrs Naudeer knew to be extremely important in the field of psychiatric nursing. She worked very closely with the staff consultants, raised the standard of nursing care and built up an impressive team.

In an interview for *Nursing Focus* in September 1982, Betty said:

> "Until I came here, I never realised quite how embroiled in bureaucracy I had become in the NHS. In recent years, it had seemed as if my days were filled with meetings. Here my responsibilities are more related to patient care. I have my own budget, and have more autonomy and more control over my working day. Obviously I have to do a certain amount of administration but the major part of my day is spent supervising patient care, which is my primary concern."

Merton, Sutton and Wandsworth Area Health Authority, which made regular inspections, were very pleased with the changes taking place. This led to The Priory's recognition by the English Nursing Board as suitable for training student nurses for the NHS. Rotations were set up with St George's, Kingston, and Long Grove Hospitals, and the arrival of learners changed the ethos of the place.

Nursing care at The Priory was earning an enviable reputation.

Renée & Camille Baudonne, Nursing Sisters
Priory Years: 1963 – 1998

Renée Baudonne had been at The Priory for 27 years when we arranged a special 10th anniversary dinner in the chapel for Dr Kelly in March 1990. At the dinner, she spoke about when she and her sister Camille first left France and came to the hospital.

> "During the first two weeks, I didn't unpack; I thought The Priory was a dreadful place. I didn't know where I was: if I'd known Heathrow was so near, I would have gone! But after that I settled down and worked for 17 years with Dr Flood.
>
> Camille and I applied to go back to France about four times but I was very much in love with The Priory. If anyone says anything bad about it I feel very hurt.
>
> It was filthy dirty back then but there was always something about the place. I suppose one day I will retire and that day I will cry, but I'm not thinking about it. We are a good team and Dr Kelly has been a very good pupil!"

It was 7 years later – by which time they had both retired (Renée after 35 years) – that I had tea with the sisters at their apartment in Surbiton.

"**Renée:** We were not married and had no children: we gave everything to The Priory. Yes, we had worries about our mother when our father died but in a way that helps, to go through somebody dying, you understand much more and can talk to people who have lost someone.

Men when they come in are very frightened, very tense. I remember going for a walk with one of the male patients and I said 'You have to let go,' and he said 'I'm not depressed, there's nothing wrong with me, I shouldn't be here.' So we just talked and when we came back he cried; he let go.

After that, men are terribly easy but to start with they are quite difficult because they don't understand that they're sick. They shouldn't be depressed or shouldn't be this or that. So to start with you have to sit and listen and let them believe they are still in charge.

When they get better they are wonderful, because they just do whatever you want them to do. Whereas we women are much more difficult, we can be hysterical, neurotic, so the difference is huge. But of course I like difficult people because I say, 'I'm going to win!'

I remember a particularly challenging patient with obsessive-compulsive disorder. He was with us while being assessed for a leucotomy[*] operation and to go into his room was to go into a sterile place. Everything was covered in white, he would only receive medication with plastic gloves on, and I was not allowed to sit down or touch anything. When he came back from his leucotomy he took me in his arms and hugged me; and when I took his blood pressure, I could touch him. That was so wonderful. I remember him more than anybody else, funnily enough.

When I first came I was looking after a patient in Room 4 and one of the psychiatrists said: 'I would give anything to be your patient, the way you look after them.' I thought, maybe I'm doing a good job! That was the first time someone complimented me. I suppose if you're a warm person and take the time to sit down with them - we were never in a hurry, you see. This is very important - not to be anxious or make patients feel you have a lot of things to do.

I was very scared once when we had a 6'3" patient with a bodyguard, on West Wing. I told the doctors we have to do something because he is getting very bad, and I was told to give him an injection.

The patient came in and the bodyguard stayed outside, and suddenly I just knew he was going to attack me. That was the first time, inside, that I felt terrible. I gave him the injection, moved away, and he followed and gave me such a punch I thought he'd broken my jaw. The nurse with me just screamed and shouted.

Afterwards, I cried of course and later went to sit on his bed and he said, 'Renée I'm very sorry...' I said 'OK, but next time just tell me in advance so I can run away!'

But we had a wonderful time and if it was to be done again I would still do it. And we met some wonderful people. Gerald Durrell, the author and zoologist, was admitted around Christmas at the end of the Sixties. He had a problem with his nose, high blood pressure and he was drinking.

Camille: He had been admitted to a hospital somewhere in London and the Ear, Nose, and Throat specialist sent him to The Priory because they thought he had an alcohol problem, which he had. So he came with his two nostrils blocked with gauze. He was scared to death; he thought he was going to die.

Renée: And he was quite depressed. But I remember talking to him (I feel that people who write are so marvellous) and he said, 'I don't like writing. I write to feed my animals; otherwise I would never do it.' He had a zoo.

---

[*] Mr Henry Marsh, the leading Neurosurgeon who carried out many Leucotomy procedures for Priory patients described it this way: "The operation is called a Stereotactic Limbic Interruption (or 'Leucotomy'). It involves making a series of very small lesions (which means a destructive hole) in a very specific part of the brain called the limbic system. The limbic system is the part of the brain that deals with emotion and arousal and the purpose of the operation is to damage the limbic system in two very small areas, thereby changing the patient's emotional balance and the level at which they become aroused and anxious."

One thing people don't understand is Electro Convulsive Therapy [ECT][*]. Once on the radio they were discussing how people shouldn't have ECT. I remember thinking *what would we do without ECT?* We have done millions, and we never had any accidents. I think if somebody is suicidal and if the tablets have only gone so far, then they have to take the chance and accept ECT.

Camille: Most doctors and nurses would have it themselves rather than the misery and despair that depression brings. ECT has saved so many from suicide.

Renée: There was a lot of anxiety when we were told The Priory was going to be sold to Americans. Some doctors and staff left, because they were frightened about what was going to happen.

Then one Saturday on the ward, Dr. Flood was not his usual self. I asked what was wrong and eventually he told me that he had a life threatening illness. I couldn't speak.

His illness was a terrible trauma for everyone, and with the Americans coming too, it was a very worrying time. Dr Kelly was there by then (he became Medical Director in the February, before Dr Flood died on the 4th July 1979) and he held meetings with all the staff.

Dr Kelly was very worried that the Americans would not honour the contracts of the staff – most of us had worked at The Priory for many years. He had a meeting with all the staff and explained the situation to us. He was going to talk to a City lawyer and a letter was written to The Priory Board, stating that the staff would support the American acquisition of The Priory provided they honoured existing contracts.

And when the Americans came, the whole atmosphere of The Priory changed: they did a very good job. You see although Dr Flood had a lot of Irish charm and was very good as a doctor, he wasn't good for business!

I didn't think Americans knew much about treatment but Mr Hughes, the man in charge, knew plenty. Later, I went to Paris with him because they wanted to open a place in France. That was very nice: he was very hard but my God he knew how to live. We were in a lovely hotel, wonderful food and wine. I was very impressed.

---

[*] ECT is a physical procedure used to treat severe, treatment-resistant depression. Electricity passes through the brain, under anaesthetic, and it is usually given in courses of six to twelve treatments. The risks relate to the anaesthetic, memory loss and confusion following treatment. Antidepressant treatment is usually started before and continued after a course of ECT. The effect seems to be similar to rebooting a computer: at some point the depressive pathways are bypassed and a normal mood takes over. For those with severe depression it can be life saving and prevent suicide.

Recent findings, discussed by Dr Allan Scott at a meeting of The Royal Society of Medicine in January 2011, show that ECT remains an important treatment, if all else fails, for intractable psychiatric illness.

Under Dr. Kelly, we had all these Registrars, whereas before we only had Drs Saeed Islam and Morven Thomson. What was very good also was to have the GP trainees, then student nurses, and finally medical students.

To be a good psychiatric nurse, you have to like people and have to have a lot of common sense. I suppose we had it. We came to England by accident and we became nurses by accident – I actually wanted to look after children. But I have enjoyed every minute of it. It's a very sad world, and you have to be strong. You mustn't cry with them, and never get involved, never."

***

I must add here that in his book *Fillets of Plaice* Gerald Durrell talks about his stay at The Priory, which he discreetly refers to as 'Abbotsford'. Describing the nurses, he said:

> "They were all in their individual ways remarkably attractive. It was rather like being looked after by the entrants for a Miss World competition. Of the day staff there was Lorraine, the Swedish blonde, whose eyes changed colour like a fiord in the sun; Zena, half English and half German, who had orange hair and completely circular and perpetually astonished blue eyes; and Nelly, a charmer from Basutoland, carved out of fine milk chocolate and with a little round nose like a brown button mushroom. Then there was the night staff. Breeda, short, blonde as honey and motherly, and, without doubt the most attractive of them all, Pimmie (a nickname derived from God knows what source) who was tall, slender and elf-like, with enormous greeny-hazel eyes the colour of a trout stream in spring. They were young and cheerful and went about their work with all the gaiety and eagerness to please of a litter of puppies.
>
> "Their gambollings were presided over by two Sisters, both French, whose combined accents would have made Maurice Chevalier sound as though he had been brought up at Oxford and had worked for the BBC for a number of years. These were the Sisters Louise [sic] and Renée and their blunt practicality in action was a pleasure to watch and to listen to."

Dr Mike McPhillips, Senior House Officer '93-'94, said of Renée:

> "Sister Renée was, even then (and she must have been in her late 50s when I was there), an impossibly glamorous woman. All the male doctors were half in love with her. She had a wonderful French charm. The way she spoke, the way she worked, the way she addressed us all. Ward Sisters like that simply don't exist anymore. Renée and Ida Durack ran Garden Wing in the old fashioned way.
>
> Then, nurses believed in the physical care of patients. They would feed them, they would help them to bed, they would consider it

their job to make sure that they slept well and that they were physically comfortable. They would hold hands with them; give them a hug or cuddle if they were stressed.

Nurses would go out to the shops for the patients – they didn't consider it demeaning or not their job or that it would cause an unhealthy collusion with the patient."

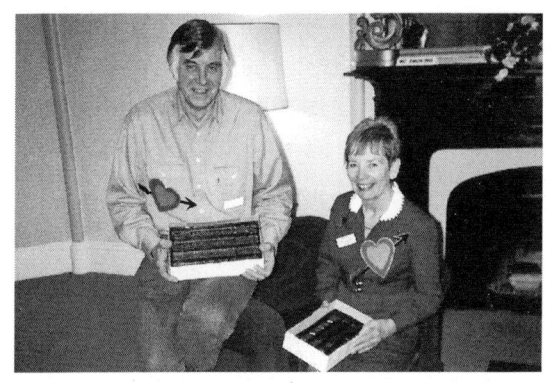

Erich Herrmann and Renée Baudonne win Mr & Ms Valentine prize, 1994

Glorianna Murphy, Nursing Sister
Priory Years: 1967 – 2003

Glorianna has been described by an ex-patient as "...one of the kindest and most fundamentally decent human beings I have ever met. She delivers compassion-based and absolutely non-judgemental nursing ministry." I think that sums her up superbly.

"I first went to The Priory as an agency nurse in 1967. After about a year, the Medical Director, John Flood asked if I'd ever thought about joining the staff. I said 'Are you asking?' He said 'Yes, I'm asking.'

So I joined on the 1st February 1968. I was in the Treatment Corridor, which was the only admission ward, with about 45 beds. Then there was Upper South, Lower South and New Wing for about 45 long stay patients. They didn't need to be cared for all the time. They came down to the dining room for meals, and had single rooms with their own furniture. The building was old, dirty and nothing was ever renewed. There was no money to spend and looking after the patients was more important than the décor.

I became one of four Sisters; there were four trained staff on the Treatment Corridor and four Sisters. The Director of Nursing, Betty Naudeer, came from Queen Mary's Hospital. It was Betty that brought student nurses to The Priory, and Dr Kelly, who was the Medical Director then, was very interested in training and was all in favour.

The thing that sticks in my mind was when Dr. Flood died. He was a very big loss. He had six children and they were like our children, because we had seen them growing up. And to see how distressed they were affected us, because we felt we had lost something too. He was already very ill and then he was stabbed one day when he went back to his house and found some intruders in his kitchen. He was sent to Queen Mary's and was there for quite a while.

In fact he came out just in time to give his daughter Marie Therese away. They actually held the wedding in The Priory grounds. He died about a month later on July 4th 1980. He was 56.

I was working on the day he died. When I was told, I went into the dining room to tell some of the staff then went over to the house to see him. Marie Claire, the youngest daughter, was very upset and was clinging on to him; she would have been about 12.

He was a popular doctor because he was so humane. Any time we had problems we went to Dr Flood, and he'd always try to help. He was not the type of person who liked argument, or to solve any big staff problems, but he was willing to listen. Unfortunately, there was no such thing as patients having to pay the fee before they left. Sometimes people paid, sometimes they didn't. That's why they had to sell a lot of The Priory grounds.

At one time we used to have extensive grounds but council houses were built there and then they had to change the outlook because the garden, as it is now, used to be the back garden. They used to have loads of trees all the way to Priory Lane. And at the end of the drive there were two houses, where the Matron and Assistant Matron lived, one on top of the other. Then they built a lot of houses. Mrs. Poole, the Medical Director's secretary was living in one of them.

The ECT room was part of the Treatment Corridor. ECT is very good for people with depression and for people who are very suicidal. It's the best treatment out. They need something to be fast. Medication can take a few weeks to work and some people are so depressed that they can't wait that long – they'd be dead. There was also the theatre, where they did the leucotomy operations. Later, of course, they went to Atkinson Morley's Hospital for the operation and back to The Priory for behaviour therapy afterwards.

Things changed as soon as the Americans bought the place. John Hughes, the Chief Executive, was really very nice. He worked hard, was always friendly and never passed by without saying something to you.

When I first arrived, I was told, 'Be very careful of the French Sisters because they are very particular about everything.' They were the main Sisters on the Treatment Corridor. I used to walk in fear! I got on all right with them but I was always very careful about what I said and did.

Renée and Camille always had Wednesdays off and at one stage I was working with a sister who decided the place wasn't all that busy so she would go to Harrods to do her shopping. So she went off early and who should she bump into in Harrods but Renée and Camille! They said 'What are you doing here? You're supposed to be working.' The next day I heard how petrified she'd been.

In fact I didn't work with Renée until the last few years but I worked with Camille for five years. I used to hear such praise about Renée from patients and used to think: *Ah! This is a person I have to look out for. I must find out how she treats patients and what's so special about her.* Renée was like a role model for me and Camille taught me a lot of things I didn't know about psychiatry.

What surprised me was how effortlessly the titled and famous mixed with the other patients. We used to have lots of lords, ladies and stars that the press never knew about, and the funny thing was that because we only had one treatment corridor they didn't mind being seen by everyone else in their worst stages and, when they recovered a little, they were happy to be moved like everyone else to the tiny recovery rooms upstairs. There used to be a coin box in the lobby and famous male singers would come out to make calls with their long hair all done up in curlers.

But being responsible for the physical and mental welfare of highly strung people could be daunting. I remember when a Hollywood film star, noted for her exuberant cleavage, had boiling water dripped on to her chest accidentally at breakfast one day. We were terrified because they were very famous breasts, insured for a lot of money, and we were scared she'd sue us, so we rushed to treat her and luckily not a mark was left.

I can't say that we like every single patient – but we tolerate them and learn to like them. Often they portray a very different picture when they arrive – they're very depressed, very anxious. You learn to get them to trust you, you give them the calmness they need, and in the end you find that they're very nice people.

I was always told that The Priory was haunted. New Wing used to be the male wing and a lot of night staff used to say they saw ghosts moving around. I never saw one myself. We had a long stay patient who killed himself one night. I had just got home, the phone rang and they asked me to go back. I went to his room on Upper West, Room 15. It was covered in blood; he had slashed his wrists with a razor blade. He died of course. But it was terrible because I knew him well and liked him. Things like that do happen in a psychiatric hospital, people do kill themselves.

There is less stigma associated with mental illness today. Most people have been depressed at one stage or another so they do understand what depression and psychiatric illness is all about. But years ago people felt that if friends or family knew that they were mentally ill, they would be scared of them.

Working at The Priory made me aware that there are a lot of people who need help and understanding. I felt that I was able to give it to them. I felt that I was able to do something to help them, both patients and staff. The staff cared for one another and I felt that I had gone into a big family. I was an only child and so I thrived on having a 'family'.

I've been lucky in that I'm very stable, both in my working life and in my mental state. I've sympathised with patients and listened to them but I don't take my work home with me.

My husband says I live for The Priory!"

***

In the early Eighties, DK inherited the Harley Street practice of a psychiatrist whose clientele largely consisted of homosexuals, transvestites and transsexuals. The doctor in question had been found dead in bed one morning. His patients were distraught and DK wasn't too happy either because the doctor's wife made him promise that he would help with the practice.

I visited the Harley Street rooms of the doctor, to meet his grieving secretary and to assess the size of his practice. Many filing cabinets were transferred to The Priory, together with a fulsome library of unusual books, which I rather enjoyed categorising.

Like most women, I rely on intuition as to a person's gender; what it is, or was, however dressed. When one of the deceased doctor's patients appeared for an appointment, I just knew he was a man dressed as a woman. Yet Dr Kelly's subsequent letter to the General Practitioner referred to 'this lady'. "She's no lady," I hazarded. "Course she is" was the rejoinder.

Imagine my glee a few days later when additional paperwork arrived: 'she' had been a Captain in the Army during the war. I tried to sustain a straight face when showing Dr Kelly the letter. "Hmm" he said, "what do you know?" When he then received a letter from the ex-Army Captain herself ...*I want you to know that I wore black lace panties for our meeting, in your honour...* that was it. From then on I was under strict instructions to refer transvestites and transsexuals to a specialist colleague.

A definite female patient around that same time felt compelled to bare her left breast whenever DK arrived on the ward. It isn't easy being a shrink.

I would try not to get upset when a patient fell off the wagon after two or three years of sobriety. It seemed so very sad – all those milestones achieved, temptations overcome, the resolve, the hopes. Yet sometimes there were more immediate considerations. Such as when an intoxicated patient tumbled through my office door and spied my shoes. "You-are-wearing..." he slurred "...red-heels! I must have you: there on the floor!" A trembling finger indicated the spot. "Right now!" he insisted, slumping into a chair. At such times, when unbefitting hilarity bubbled up, I mustered any scrap of dignity I could find.

Patients arrived in many ways. The famous might be led in via a side door and secreted up back stairs to the doctor's office. Or someone rather manic might turn up in a just-purchased spanking new Rolls Royce: the buy of a high. When two judges were admitted during the same week, with all the potential embarrassment of beak to beak recognition, I had to make sure their paths never crossed. And I could tell instantly what mood one patient was in because my door would swing open and he would pose with a rose between his teeth. Such moments were most welcome when things got heavy.

I took great pride in being on top of DK's outpatient accounts, with very few non-payers, and he was more than happy to leave it to me. I did once mention a reminder I had prepared. It was to a patient with gangster associations; someone he had been persuaded to see against his better judgement. DK went a whiter shade of pale and declared: "You are *absolutely forbidden* to send a reminder: to hell with your pride!"

It was an irony that whilst we Priory staff did all we could to protect a patient's confidentiality, they often blew it themselves. I was phoned one day by a patient's helicopter pilot, to request that a large white sheet be placed on the front lawn; minutes later the 'copter duly descended. It seems likely that all around, including the children scaling the boundary wall to relish the spectacle, spotted the family name emblazoned on the helicopter's sides.

Another example of a patient blowing his own cover came in the mid-Eighties when DK had a long discussion with a just-admitted nobleman about the best pseudonym for him during his stay. He returned to see him again later in the day, only to find him on his mobile to the *Daily Mail*. He had contacted Nigel Dempster to tell him about his 'nervous exhaustion'. The result was an exposé about his alcoholism and DK blamed himself for not confiscating his phone.

When I learned that the Archbishop of Westminster, Cardinal Basil Hume was to visit a patient, I thought *how on earth can I hope to disguise him? Whatever his attire, his revered and kindly face and that unmistakeable shock of hair will give him away.* But he had absolutely no intention of being incognito. He swept in, resplendent in full regalia, clearly relishing the admiration received and the words exchanged with patients along the way.

Some patients had famous other halves and they would tend to make late appointments so that their partner could avoid curious glances in the waiting room. Or they could wait in my office and avoid it that way. One rock star came with several significant others - the rest of the band. They took the office over in fact, commandeered the phone and sprawled about generally.

There was another scenario – what should you do when, as someone who worked at The Priory, you bumped into patients in a social setting? It could be very awkward. I always left it to them: if they wanted to acknowledge me, fine. But there was this wretched stigma attached to psychiatry and people didn't want to be associated with it. Obviously the last thing we staff were going to do was march up to them and talk about The Priory. Still, you couldn't blame them for being sensitive.

One evening I had two engagements in town. At a wine bar in Knightsbridge, I was having a drink with an old friend and noticed an outpatient at the bar with a chap. She and I exchanged discreet smiles. Later in the evening, I was astounded to see the same lady walk through the door of the restaurant in Mayfair where I was having dinner with another friend. She too was with a different fellow. Barely able to contain our mirth, we managed to visit the ladies simultaneously and agreed that if we'd seen this in a sitcom it would have seemed contrived.

Yet another scenario is experiencing the stigma within oneself. I was off work for a week shortly before Christmas one year and much to my embarrassment I bumped into one of our Visiting Consultants, Glyn Davies. I was at the local shop getting milk and he came in. He took one look at me and said, "You haven't got flu: you're depressed." My inner critic felt terribly ashamed. It was all right for others to be human but not me. After all, I worked in a place where people were *really* depressed and I should be there doing my bit.

As for being a psychiatrist out and about socially, DK found that it wasn't always wise to admit to being a shrink. If he did, he could find himself stuck with someone determined to take advantage of his expertise. So when his antenna suggested it would be prudent, he told them instead that he was a venereologist. This left him free to tuck into the canapés very peacefully!

Most days, journalists in the national papers vied with each other to find new ways to describe The Priory. It was a 'white fairytale palace', 'a haven', a 'chocolate box'. *They should try working here*, I'd think on a bad day. *It might look like a chocolate box but the selection inside is predominantly nutty.* No, I preferred a patient's description, when he booked in to escape Christmas each year: "Here I am again, at my zany country club."

Setting off home I would sometimes look back at those secretive walls and dramatic spires. For a couple of years, the sharp-eyed could spy an owl amongst the spires. It was plastic; it twirled on a pole and was designed to scare off pigeons. But Steve the Falconer, who became a regular visitor, was far more effective. I think patients mistook him for one of them, as he strutted around, a hooded falcon on his arm. Not many would see him clamber through high windows, release his falcon and banish pigeon squatters.

5
Trail Blazing Academy:
Research, Academic and Educational Links with the NHS

Of all Desmond Kelly's trail blazing plans, perhaps the most ambitious was to build up a teaching tradition that would not only strengthen the hospital's clinical standards but would also raise its academic reputation.

In October 1976, when The Priory was inspected by the Royal College of Psychiatrists, it was given provisional approval to train Registrars. The in-house Registrars at the time were Drs Saeed Islam and Morven Thomson.

The next inspection was due in June 1982, by which time Saeed was a Priory Consultant and Morven was a Consultant at Sutton General Hospital. The criteria for these inspections had become far more rigorous and even Dr Thomas Bewley, the Dean of the College was involved.

The current Registrar, Dr Michael Rowlands, had been in post since November 1981, working under 7 staff consultants and 12 Visiting Consultants. Dr Renate Hauser, a Research Registrar from Basle University in Switzerland, was due to start in August 1982 and an advertisement had been placed for yet another Registrar.

To give an idea of patient numbers, during 1981 there were 625 acute admissions at The Priory. There were 67 acute beds for general psychiatry (to be increased to 82 in September 1982 as part of the remodelling planned by John Hughes); 26 psychogeriatric beds and 21 beds for alcoholism at Galsworthy House nearby.

The Clinical Tutor was Dr Timothy Sicks, a charming Canadian, and one of the psychiatrists who had interviewed me. I loved the way he popped into my office when passing "to see how you are", but taking the opportunity to check out his good looks in the mirror or tweak an eyebrow. Dr Sicks took his teaching responsibilities very seriously and he and DK had prepared assiduously for this all-important inspection. In a memo to Desmond, Tim was confident:

> "...When I look through the file I see a welter of memos between me and you that reflect a great deal of thought about Registrar training. It seems to me that The Priory has a great deal to offer, and that we have given Dr Rowlands a very good deal. We have to stand or fall on that."

Someone was plainly impressed with the improved facilities: Professor Sir Desmond Pond, a former President of the Royal College of Psychiatrists (1978-1981). For in May 1982, a month before the College inspection, Sir Desmond joined The Priory's teaching staff. It was a considerable coup to capture such an eminent authority.

Sir Desmond had also been a professor at the London Hospital (1966-1982) and was still Chief Scientist to the Department of Health and Social Security. One of his most influential positions was as Chairman of the Conference of Medical Royal Colleges and Faculties, the first psychiatrist to enjoy the distinction.

Sir Desmond Pond chaired the Thursday morning Clinical Meetings once a fortnight and Desmond Kelly chaired the other Thursdays. Meetings were attended by the consultants, registrars, nurses, pharmacist, occupational therapists, visiting doctors and medical students. It was a time for the most challenging inpatients to be discussed. Sir Desmond would have interviewed the patient beforehand, then at the meeting itself the registrar would outline the history and Sir Desmond would talk to the patient in front of the assembled company.

Everyone would put forward their ideas for further treatment options and the whole process was of great help to the patient's consultant. The patient, too, realised that receiving the combined wisdom of such a multi-disciplinary gathering was a bonus. The clinical part of the meeting would be followed by a general discussion of current issues.

By 1985 The Priory had forged links with several teaching hospitals and begun funding research posts at the Middlesex and Charing Cross Hospitals, while paying for junior doctors from those hospitals to spend a six-month placement at The Priory. Four posts were created for registrars who would gain special experience in the treatment of eating disorders and drug and alcohol abuse at The Priory, under the supervision of the consultants.

The experiment was so successful that the teaching programme was extended to trainee GPs and nurses. And after the Royal College of General Practitioners and the English Nursing Board had given it their blessing, nursing rotations were set up with St George's, Kingston, and Long Grove hospitals.

It was a terrible shock for us all when Sir Desmond Pond died of cancer in June 1986. His wisdom, humour and gentle ways were summed up perfectly in his obituary in The British Medical Journal:

> "...He expressed his personality lightly in manner and dress: his informal jacket and peaked cap suited him and were certainly daring in a medical academic. Attractive, perpetually youthful, and even tempered, he had great personal charm, an attribute that seems under-rated these days, yet it enabled him to work constructively with an astonishing variety of people. It is sad that his retirement is so brief..."

In 1991, batches of medical students from University College Hospital and the Middlesex Hospital began to arrive on six-week placements to prepare for their clerkship in psychiatry. Later that year, The Priory was granted an official seal of approval as a teaching institution when Dr Kelly was appointed Visiting Professor of Psychiatry to University College Medical School, the first and only such appointment of a private-sector psychiatrist.

As you will hear from Dr Mike McPhillips, one of the junior doctors at the time, the transition from overcrowded, under-funded NHS hospitals to the comparative luxury of The Priory was something of a culture shock for the young trainees, many of whom disapproved of private medicine.

***

Excerpt from a letter written to my sister Susan in America, 27/6/85

> "...Dr Kelly went to lecture in Russia at the beginning of June. Although he had been invited by the Soviet Institute of Psychiatry, the Russian Consulate gave us terrible trouble getting the visa. I ended up at the Consulate one Saturday morning and spent more than three hours trying not to be provoked by their hostility. Several people told me to go away but I wouldn't budge. I was so persistent I amazed myself.
>
> At one point, the Consulate sent me to the Embassy and miraculously the gate was open so I marched right in to where a group of men were talking. I headed for the one who looked most influential to seek his help and was immediately surrounded by three heavies! Only later did I find out (from a diplomatic cop outside who had been watching the proceedings), that I had selected the Ambassador himself. Eventually, I got to see the Head of the Consular section. I think DK was grateful for my efforts, without which he wouldn't have got to Russia. He went to the Bolshoi Ballet too. Rotter."

Dr Bill Shanahan, Registrar
Priory Year: 1987

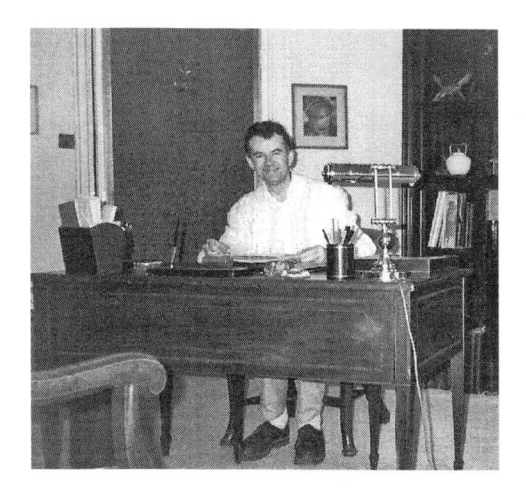

Now Medical Director at the Capio Nightingale Hospital in Marylebone, Bill Shanahan relates how his year as a junior doctor at The Priory changed his life. This photograph, taken on the quiet in Dr Thompson's office, was supplied by Bill. He describes it as '...like a child putting on his father's shoes!' Bill's medical directorship of the Capio Nightingale Hospital proves that he is more than big enough to fill them.

"The situation in Ireland was terrible for jobs and what they'd done (a bit of an Irish solution to an Irish problem) was they'd frozen all the posts so that consultants were going to work in Canada and various places and there was no movement anywhere unless you knew somebody. So I thought I'd like a break and the UK beckoned.

I qualified [gained Membership of The Royal College of Psychiatrists] in 1986. And because in Ireland the NHS hospitals are attached to private hospitals and I had done my pre-membership days in a private hospital, it seemed quite a reasonable step to come here and do the same thing.

So I applied at The Priory. I met Desmond and Peter Storey [Visiting Consultant at The Priory 1987-1991, and Second Opinion Consultant after Sir Desmond Pond died] for lunch and got asked some very basic questions. I thought *what are they asking that for?* But it was to establish that I actually had some credentials! There was a sense of 'why exactly does this man with membership want to work in The Priory without taking a senior post?' Was I some sort of impostor?! I explained that I wanted the job to get a foothold in the UK, which in fact is what it gave me. Because through that job and through John Cobb's [Consultant Psychiatrist at The Priory] connections with the Maudsley, I met Ian Falloon [community-based psychiatrist in Buckinghamshire, with connections to the University of Oxford], which gave me my research year in Buckingham, from which I got my publications, from which I got my Charing Cross Hospital post!

At first it was quite difficult for me at The Priory because I was with people who were on the Charing Cross rotation, which meant that these guys were guaranteed work and I wasn't. But it was very good for me to see the work they were doing. It was them that made me realise that if I didn't get anything substantial I would probably have to leave the private sector anyway and go and do some locum work just to get known. The great thing about working in the UK was that, by and large, most of the jobs were open to the best candidate. And I got a good job at Charing Cross with my papers, even though I had done my basic work only at The Priory. But I had huge support from Priory Consultants – Desmond, Saeed Islam and David Thompson were particularly supportive.

It was extraordinary to meet all these huge people in psychiatry whose papers I'd been reading the year before. There they all were at The Priory: Alec Coppen, Peter Storey, Will Sargant, the great authors of the day. Will Sargant was wonderful, fascinating, and we were in conversation one night at dinner. It was marvellous! These were opportunities you'd never get in a small country like Ireland. What I also liked was Peter Storey's ability to align neurology with psychiatry, so his grand rounds [clinical meetings] were fabulous. He would look at the neurological aspects of a case and you'd get that whole feeling of medicine back in psychiatry. And there was Professor Sir Desmond Pond, Tim Sicks, Gerald Libby. I liked being able to present my own cases to those grand rounds, being allowed to demonstrate what I could do.

It was all in a day's work when I had to repatriate a patient who wasn't very well. He thought he was going back to Australia but in fact he was going to Stockholm and I got the job of taking him on the plane. He was sedated and I had a little bag of tablets in case he came to too quickly, because of course we wanted him to remain sedated on the plane. A couple of security guards sat nearby.

The Captain wanted to know if I had any particular instructions, and I said 'Yes, you mustn't mention Stockholm!' So when the plane took off, they made their announcement and ended, 'and it's 5 degrees... where we're going'. People sat up and looked around; the patient came to slightly and said, 'What's going on?' I said, go back to sleep. Later, the voice came up again '... pleased to tell you that the sun is shining ... at our destination.' People were thinking *what is this pilot on about?!* It all worked out OK in the end but it was funny.

My room was in Priory-owned flats on the main road there – the junior doctors had two rooms – Richard Allison [another Registrar] had one with his wife, and I had the other. The flat above me was given over to the parents of patients and one night somebody must have come in a little intoxicated because the next thing was that my bedroom door shot open and there was this mother, who asked what I was doing in her bedroom?! I thought *it isn't going to go down very well if this gets out.* I had to quickly call the porter and get the lady escorted upstairs. She was so drunk she didn't remember a thing about it. They changed the locks after that.

People had told me, 'You'll see Richmond Park, it's very handy.' Well I didn't expect Richmond Park to go past my window, which it duly did that October, because it was the big wind of 1987 when about 100,000 trees went past the window of the flat! They were exciting times because the same year Stephen Roche, an Irishman, won the Tour de France, so the Irish were riding high! And I got introduced to cricket, through Saeed Islam's fascination with the game.

The upper middle class patients, the people I almost expected to be difficult, were absolutely charming, delighted to be helped and very grateful. And once you got them going you could banter with them and they were very funny. The last thing they wanted was any ceremony.

By contrast, there were a few people who were very distressed over business deals that had gone wrong, and of course I heard their take on it. I remember believing implicitly in their innocence and then got a great shock to find out on two occasions that they were not innocent at all!

Late, unexpected admissions didn't happen very often and the reality is that you might get out at 3am and kick the bed a few times but once you get into the room with the patient, you change completely. The great thing about being a junior is that you build up a quick rapport with the patient. Often, they tell you things that they won't tell the consultant for quite some time. I've realised that in subsequent years with my own trainees. Patients really want to make a bond with somebody and you're the first person through the door.

If there was a down side, it was that the families of patients wouldn't take the juniors seriously. You could work really hard and then they'd ring up and abuse you on the telephone and want to speak to the consultant. They often came back and apologised later, in fairness, but when you were stressed it wasn't very nice, particularly on a Sunday evening when you had worked very hard with a patient and were told you were not being helpful. I remember one person kept telling me that I was 'very wishy-washy'! The consultants explained that anxious people take it out on the junior staff. It was a good lesson actually because I've seen it subsequently. When people are getting nervous about their family members they always get cross and you have to accommodate that, its part of your learning.

It was chance – serendipity - that I got into the addiction side of things. There was a huge addiction unit where I trained in Dublin and although I didn't work there I was on call for it and remember going up and seeing people who were very reluctant to be admitted, and talking them into staying and realising I could do it. That gives you a real sense of achievement, that you can make someone realise they need help, where they didn't see it before, breaking down that initial resistance.

At The Priory there was the Galsworthy unit, where again I didn't work, but occasionally I'd be on call. Then by chance my first job at Charing Cross was with the first consultant in addictions there, Brian Wells. So I became the first trainee in West London in addictions.

I think I have a way (without being conceited about it) of making people feel that they're not cornered anymore. I don't criticise. My approach is – this is very difficult, you're feeling guilty, full of remorse and fed up with fingers wagging at you from the corner. There is hope, change is possible, and unlike lots of other conditions this is not a death sentence. The prognosis may actually be bad today but very good tomorrow. It's not a tumour: we can actually stop it. We may not be able to cure it but we can give you back everything else.

It's almost like a child who has been visited by all of the good fairies at the crib side and given lots of qualities and attributes. But then the alcoholic fairy comes along and realises she can't take everything back but she can inject something that will stop the others working. So it actually poisons you. And if you take away the substance, all the other qualities can rise again. I like the feeling of instilling hope and that change is possible. Also I like the fact that I have had bin men do very well and judges not do very well, and vice versa, so you don't know where you're going to get your successes from. Everyone can make it.

Even people who were so badly knocked off that they had pretty bad Alzheimer-like dementia, have done well. I remember a high court judge repeatedly telling me he wasn't an alcoholic and getting off the bed and walking into the wardrobe instead of out the door.

What I've managed to do through literary allusion and metaphor is to let people map their life stories. I can pick a book they know, or a movie they've seen and give them imagery within that to show their own journey a little bit. Or quote a line from a poem – someone as deep as Gerard Manley Hopkins, who talks about depression wonderfully, or Yeats, or even Yogi Berra – 'if you come to a fork in the road, take it.'

When people come to you they expect nothing but bad news – medicine, liver problems, jaundice, and if you can take them away for a while into that little world of make believe or fiction and get them to remember fictional characters, they forget that they're sick. For two or three minutes you might float them above the rough seas of sickness and their loss of health and the failure of hope; bring them somewhere that might relax the mind. But then you've got to get back to the therapy because they'll happily distract you from the fact that they're drinking a bottle of whisky a day.

What's amazing is that I've been able to tell you so much about just one year. No other year has yielded so many memories, had such variety and been so important."

Dr Shanahan's last anecdote earns the title **Gunning for Margaret**

"I looked after somebody who I met about four years later at Harry's Bar in Venice, where she was having lunch with Margaret Thatcher. I was sitting at a table with a friend and noticed lots of people surrounding another table. I thought they were getting extraordinary attention and then I spotted this person with Mrs Thatcher. She gave me a little nod. Of course with psychiatric patients you're terrified that they might not want to be recognised but as she had, in effect, said hello, I thought I was on good grounds to go over. When I stood up, the people at the table nearby turned out to be bodyguards who thought I was going to attack! They had listened to our Irish accents throughout lunch and we almost got set upon by these people! There was a little flurry of rapid movement just to clarify what we were all going to do. So that was an interesting afternoon. I had wondered what the big bulges were in their pockets. Guns!"

***

In February 1990, a Priory Research Symposium was held [see Seminar Listing at the end of the book], when eight of the brightest and most talented young doctors of their generation came together to present their research at London Teaching Hospitals during their tenure as Priory Research Fellows.

Professor Rachel Rosser, Head of the Department of Psychiatry, University College and Middlesex School of Medicine said:

> "The Priory provides an extraordinary model at both the academic and service level. Dr John Cobb, Clinical Tutor to the Fellows, paid tribute to "the great achievement of Dr Kelly in creating a teaching hospital atmosphere in a private hospital and the very high standards of the junior staff on the rotation scheme. This cost The Priory Hospitals Group £100,000, on research, mostly in the public sector. Fellows Day was ample proof of money well spent."

By 1991 the teaching reputation of The Priory was so excellent that Professor Rosser had a suggestion to make: medical students from University College Hospital and The Middlesex should undertake part of their clerkship in psychiatry at The Priory. This was to be an outstanding success and by October 1994, 86 medical students had passed through The Priory's doors. In the previous three years their tutor, Dr Jeanie Speirs, had done fine work with them.

Dr Mike McPhillips, Senior House Officer
Priory Years: 1993 - 1994

"Thinking back to my first days at The Priory, I was slightly intimidated to be there at all. It had quite a reputation as a glamorous place where celebrities and well-known people were treated. I had done many years of NHS practice and didn't know anything about private medicine but I did have an inkling that it would be smart.

I was going to work with a chap called David Craggs. He was running the addictions unit and I was aware that it worked in a very different way from anything available in the NHS. It was an abstinence based treatment with a 12-step programme.

The Priory was a place very much dominated by the Consultants. In the NHS, the man who knows the most is probably seeing the fewest patients and supervising a team of junior doctors who actually do most of the work. In the private sector it's precisely the opposite; the patients and all of the staff really hang on the presence or absence of the Consultant.

One of my earliest memories was the Monday medical lunch, a very formal affair. It was held in the chapel and again was dominated by the Consultants. But I hadn't eaten many meals in a chapel and I wasn't used to breaking bread in the presence of my Consultant!

Later, I came to think of The Priory almost as a finishing school. The people skills and clinical skills of the Consultants were superior; they handled people incredibly well. And I guess you would if your profession is looking after people who are demanding, entitled, and mentally ill.

It made me realise that most of the behaviour I had seen towards patients in NHS hospitals – by consultants, doctors, nurses, gardeners, waiters, porters

– was just rude by comparison with the way people were treated at The Priory.

It made me realise that even on my most polite day I was actually a bit brash, perhaps a bit tactless. Relentlessly working in a system that's based on rationing access to services hardens you. You get used to saying 'no' a lot and that blocks a psychiatric relationship.

One of the things the private sector does par excellence is level the playing field: the patient is powerful. If they don't like the advice they get or the way it's delivered, they simply see another doctor (who is only too glad to have your patient).

At The Priory, each of us was assigned to a Consultant but we also looked after general patients within the hospital. So half of my time was spent serving Galsworthy Lodge and being the specialist Senior House Officer (SHO) attached to that unit. The other half of my time was spent in the main hospital looking after depressed, anxious, obsessive or post-traumatically distressed patients.

I was seeing patients I'd only read about in text books, because these patients barely existed in the NHS. If you were looking after inpatients in the NHS you were looking after people who came in under a Section 2 or Section 3 [of the Mental Health Act] and who were incredibly ill. Whereas, I began to encounter for the first time people who were simply depressed, simply anxious, simply suffering with obsessive-compulsive disorder (OCD) or other psychiatric complaints I'd only ever seen in outpatients before. So I was catching them at an acute phase of their illness when they were ill enough to be in hospital and I was seeing how they were treated. It was absolutely fascinating and wonderful learning material.

Galsworthy Lodge was a very alien experience. It seems very odd nowadays, when I've spent my career in abstinence work and around the 12-step approach, but the entire language, culture and conduct of 12-step therapy was a complete shock to me. I didn't understand a word anybody said. It seemed monumentally unscientific and incredibly 'de-skilling', because the very first thing they wanted to do in Galsworthy Lodge was to get patients *off* all medication. Probably the only qualification I had – as I knew nothing about their psychotherapy – was to put people *on* medication! So the first thing they taught me to do was start talking and stop prescribing.

It was an option to sit in on groups. We were pretty busy as SHOs and so one of the constant laments of my colleagues was that I really should take part in the programme or learn more about the therapy but I spent my whole time clerking patients. In those days, the education of doctors was something you did out of hours. If you wanted to take part you had to give up your lunch or come in early or stay late. That was the received culture. Junior doctors worked incredibly hard and I spent a great deal of time running around writing up drug cards, admitting and discharging patients, composing essays to GPs, chasing x-ray results, going on Consultants' clinical rounds, going on my own clinical rounds and talking to nurses. So there wasn't a lot of time to be going to therapy groups.

But 9 to 5 didn't exist for an ambitious young doctor. The only way you were going to get post-graduate education was to work well beyond the hours recommended. I put in a lot of hours at The Priory at nights, weekends, when I was on call, in my supposed breaks; I was in the library or in the therapy programme or learning. That was how you got on: that was expected.

To help local GPs and Consultants, The Priory established a 24-hour emergency scheme, which meant they could call at any time for advice, assessments or home visits. I didn't encounter the worried well; they barely existed. In terms of foolish prior prejudices, I had imagined that the patients wouldn't be very ill. But nobody wants to be an inpatient in a psychiatric hospital, luxurious or not.

When the private sector is spoken of within the public sector, those who don't know anything about it imagine that private doctors spend half their time on the golf course. They're shocked to discover the sort of hours that private doctors work, which are incredibly long, I'll vouch. And that the illnesses they're dealing with are as bad if not worse than anything you see within the NHS.

At The Priory, junior doctors had a very jolly time. Four of us were on training schemes and were going to be psychiatrists and the other four were GP trainees doing a psychiatric job to boost their psychiatric experience. We helped each other out a lot, ate and socialised together and talked about the various stresses and strains together. The hours were long, the work was tough but wherever you went you got a biscuit and a cup of tea. You were aware that this was as good as it got. I really believed I was working in the finest private hospital in the United Kingdom.

Dr Kelly had just become Professor Kelly, and we referred to him as that. This was a hospital conscious of its traditions and everyone rapidly learned that Professor Kelly had developed a lot of this, such as my own job - the attachment to the Charing Cross Psychiatric Training Scheme was his innovation. He made the link with St George's and created a Priory Research Fellowship. There was a Research Fellow from St George's in the Eating Disorders Unit. These were things that Desmond had created and was proud of and they were highly innovative at the time. My own job was a complete anomaly within the NHS. I knew of no other psychiatrist who had the opportunity to work, as an NHS employee, in a private hospital.

I then went on to copy it – creating something similar with Billy Shanahan. It was, and remains, a very good idea where both services have something to offer each other.

I had chafed as a junior hospital doctor under the informal (unwritten) but definite dress code of white coat doctor. Psychiatry struck me as having a different dress code. It was very plain that psychiatrists could express themselves so they wore a huge range of clothing, from Oscar Wilde outfits to training shoes and t-shirts.

My act of rebellion was to grow my hair. And if I say so myself, it was a rather splendid, thick and lustrous ponytail that hung in a great snake down my back. I was 30 years of age and was sitting for post-graduate exams, a very earnest affair. You have to examine a patient in front of Consultants. I had cherished this beautiful ponytail and was aware that I had the wretched exam coming up for Membership of the Royal College of Psychiatrists. I knew that I had to put on a suit and pretend to be like a Consultant and I couldn't possibly do that with my ponytail.

With immense regret on holiday in Thailand I went into a villainous barber, who swore that he had trained in Carnaby Street and he took my beautiful ponytail right off in one fell swoop. I brought it home in a shoe box and kept it for years.

Of course when I came back people didn't recognise me, and I went to take my exam and passed. I've always held the view that you do dress for success a bit. If you dress in an odd way you create unnecessary difficulties.

The Consultants had been angelic about it because it was quite evident that they were surprised when I first arrived. They would look at my hair and would think of saying something about it but then talk about something else. They were psychiatrists of course. I think a cardiologist would have taken me to one side and said 'My boy, if you're hoping to rise in this profession you might like to look the part.' But plenty told me afterwards. People were congratulating me all over the hospital – 'Oh, it looked *awful*!'

The staff contained hearty, warm, rounded people. Take Virginia the Pharmacist. Virginia wasn't simply handing things over the counter in the Pharmacy, she was very much on the wards, talking to patients and doctors and making sure everybody was doing the right thing!

What Desmond managed to communicate was a sense of unashamed elitism. And of course in your own heart you wanted one day to be thought of like that, as wise and eminent, modest and able. He was a very impressive leader of men and it just flowed down through the hospital. I learnt so much walking around in his wake and that of David Craggs.

It was all downhill from there! I had to go back to the NHS, it nearly broke my heart. It wasn't long before I began to think of going back to the private sector. The Priory had got under my skin. I went back as a Consultant in 2002."

In August 1995 those responsible for medical student training wrote to Dr Jeanie Speirs:

> "The Priory has been uniformly rated as invaluable. The survey of

> undergraduate placements indicated that students marked your firm as excellent, very good and good in all modalities..."

By 1997, The Royal Free and University College Medical School were linked and the RFUCMS medical students rated The Priory Hospital the best psychiatry teaching firm of 1997/98. They were to confirm their endorsement for the following years, 1998/99.

Other departments were training nurses, therapists and psychologists for the NHS, and our research registrars worked at St George's, Charing Cross and other teaching hospitals. We were proud that the private and public sectors were able to work together in the best interests of patients.

A total of 50 doctors/medical students in London were receiving some part of their clinical psychiatric training at The Priory Hospital each year.

The Royal College carried out regular approval visits, when they reviewed the standards of clinical practice, the environment, and the academic programme. The hospital's academic links helped to maintain a high clinical standard and underlined Roehampton Priory Hospital's national reputation in acute psychiatric treatment and care.

The training/academic posts at the hospital:

Two Senior House Officers on the Charing Cross rotation scheme, based at the hospital on a rolling nine month placement; one Senior House Officer from University College London's psychiatric training scheme had a six monthly rotation at the hospital (commenced 1996); St George's Hospital Medical School had two part-time psychiatry fellows working at the hospital for 12 months of their research period; two GP trainees spent six month attachments at the hospital on an ongoing basis, and Royal Free and University College Medical School had medical student clinical psychiatric placements – four students were attached to clinical teams for four week periods during term time (commenced 1991).

By the middle of 1991, with his 21st birthday coming up, I thought about my son obsessively. Was he happy? Did he hate me? Did he even think about me? Was he dead?

A letter marked private and confidential plopped through the door as I was leaving for The Priory on the 13th June that year. Intrigued, I opened it there and then. It was the adoption agency. No, it was an aberration. This is what comes of wanting something too much, I told myself, *your mind is playing tricks.* And yet as I read the lines again and again they still looked real.

"...I am pleased to let you know that I have recently been contacted by your son, Robert, who is making enquiries regarding his background. I have been able to tell him that you have previously contacted us and he has asked me as a first step to write to you on his behalf..."

Just a few words, swimming in and out of focus; words I had waited 19 years to read. My shaking fingers dialled my friend Sheila. "It's happened!" I cried the moment she picked up. She knew the agonies I had been going through and immediately realised what this meant. We agreed that I was far too emotional to call the agency myself, so Sheila would do it for me as soon as their offices opened. She would tell them of my ecstatic, enfeebled condition and that I would phone later in the day.

I should mention that not many people knew about this secret from my past, just family and a few close friends. And having worked with Dr Kelly for 9 years by then, I had confided in him, for who can be easier to talk to than a psychiatrist? But I had agonised over the years about how open I should be with people about this huge part of my past. How could I hope to explain with any clarity a decision I had made when so young; a decision so complex and confusing that I couldn't make sense of it myself? They would probably judge me (I did more than enough of that for myself); they might even pity me or look down on me as a harlot. Whatever their reaction, telling them would churn up emotions I had learned to control.

I don't know if I seemed normal as I went about my business that momentous morning but at least it was a Thursday so the consultants were safely out of the way at their clinical meeting. By about noon I felt composed enough to call the agency. Instead of phoning from my office, where I would doubtless be disturbed, I shut myself into an empty consultant's room.

I got through to Rose, the social worker who had written to me. She explained how Robert had made an appointment to see her and was 'amazed and extremely pleased' to be presented with my 1987 letter. He certainly hadn't expected anything so positive and felt enormously encouraged.

She described him as tall, slim and good looking, with curly fair hair. I was a bit anxious when she said that he'd had a 'stormy and prolonged adolescence'. But she assured me that she found him to be considerate and thoughtful.

Rose suggested that I should write a letter to Robert, via the agency, enclosing a photograph. 'Keep it light and newsy', she said, 'tell him about yourself now; don't go into long explanations about the past'. He would then write back. My boy would write back! I went for a long walk in Richmond Park that evening, where I hugged trees and whispered an old familiar mantra: 'I'm a Mum, I'm a Mum.'

Back home I began my light and newsy letter.

> "Dear Robert, It's hard to believe that I'm writing this letter and even harder to know what to say. It would be impossible, too, to describe my feelings when I opened the letter from the agency. Perhaps absolute joy will do for starters…"

Rose promised that as soon as his answer arrived, she would phone me. I would collect his letter from her office because waiting for the post was unthinkable. When she called on the 25th June I dashed into Dr Kelly's office. "The adoption people say there's a letter waiting for me!" "Off you go then!" he beamed, "Go now!"

I drove to the agency as fast as I could but it was raining hard, the lights were all red and there were too many damned cars in the way. When I burst through the agency's door, Rose was there to meet me. I have no idea what she said – my entire focus was on a large envelope in her hand.

She was really sweet and I knew I should concentrate but I just wanted to be alone with that envelope. At last I escaped and ran through the rain to the car and to my son.

The large item was a birthday card. How had he known it was my birthday? Perhaps he knew all sorts of things about me now? Next I saw his *photograph. Just head and shoulders and taken at a distance, but it was my baby all grown up.*

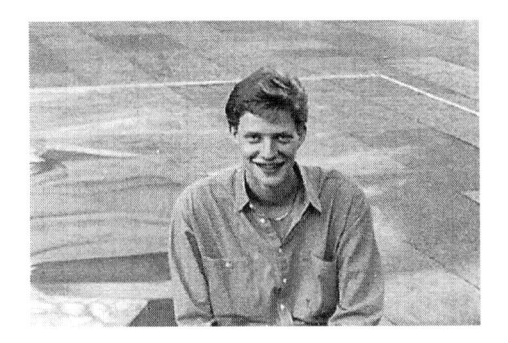

Then I read his letter.

> "Dear Dorothy, I am thrilled to be writing this letter to you, knowing you'll be reading it in a few days. I hope you are in good health and enjoying life. If your photographs are anything to go by, then you certainly look as if you are. I received your letter last Wednesday, your 39th birthday. It was a very special day – I achieved nothing at work! There I had, in my hand, a letter and photos from you to me - it was exhilarating – and I must say you don't look 39, I'm proud! It seems you lead a very active life – we certainly have things in common – I love the sound of the wine-tasting weekend! ..."

He went on to describe the jobs he'd had – for example as a chef in a jazz restaurant - and about his love of music, particularly Pink Floyd and Led Zeppelin. He ended with:

"…I now look forward to seeing you, hopefully in the near future. I am *so so* glad you got in touch with the agency…"

I pored over these treasures, such tangible proof of my 20 year old son. And I was glad to be parked in a quiet road, my hankie the sole confidant of my tears.

6
Maintaining the Fabric

What was The Priory *really* like? This chapter contains the memories of some of the men and women who kept the hospital functioning at a fundamental level. Be warned: their reflections can be earthy.

Bobbie was 79 at the time we met up at her home in Somersham, Cambridgeshire. An enthusiastic member of her local dance club, she was a petite, spry figure who spoke fondly of her years at The Priory. I had taken Doris Day the tea lady with me, to spark Bobbie's memories. But she needed no prompting and had made diligent notes beforehand.

Laura (Bobbie) Gray Milk Maid/Linen Lady
Priory Years: 1951 - 1983

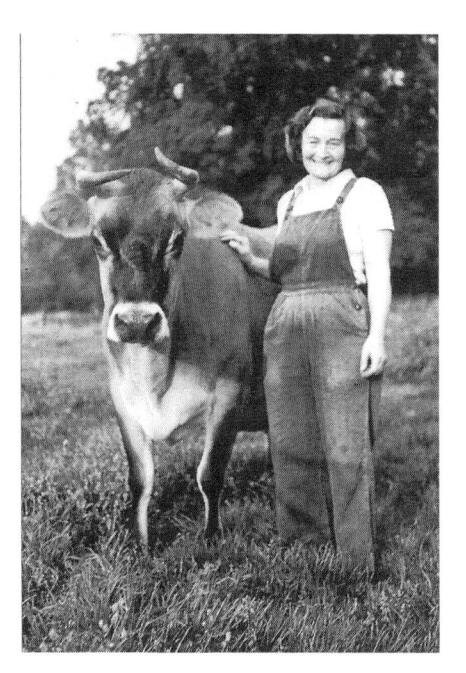

"I joined The Priory at the end of 1951. They needed a hand milker. I had been in the Land Army during the war and that was where I was taught to kill and skin a rabbit and get it ready for the table. I found my diploma the other day: Women's Land Army Proficiency Certificate, October 1945.

"This is to certify that Miss L Bradley has been awarded a proficiency badge. Milking and dairy work and has gained Distinction."

That's what I like: Distinction! The week I joined up all my hair had to come off. Chestnut, it was. After the war I worked with ponies at the Festival of Britain but when that folded I needed a job. My aunt saw an advertisement The Priory had placed in the Barnes Herald.

When I went for the interview I was taken above the stables to what was to be my room. There were cobwebs up the stairs and grit and muck – nobody had been up there for years. No furniture, nothing. I wrote and refused the job and had a letter straight back from Dr Brown [Medical Superintendent], who said would you please come and let *me* interview you. So I went and was shown another room they had prepared and I was very pleased. Even though it was on the 'Top Treatment Corridor' (I didn't know what that meant) and up 50 steps. There was no heating at The Priory then, other than coal fires in every room but I was given six bundles of wood a week. The nurses or domestics had to do the fireplaces early, probably when the patients were having breakfast.

I didn't know why I was given a pass key to get to my room, or that there was a patient in the next room, and I certainly didn't know that it was a psychiatric hospital. I just knew they wanted somebody to milk cows and work under Ted the Herdsman.

The Priory's farm was about 50 acres and when I joined there were 10 hand milking cows, 6 calves, and chickens.

We kept The Priory going with milk and chickens and the Head Gardener kept it going with vegetables. I carried the milk around on yokes, which went around the neck and had 5 gallon buckets hanging off each side. Although we were still on rations following the war, I was allowed a pint of milk a day because I worked on the land.

There was a milking shed, a dairy, a cowshed long enough to have storage for straw and hay, and an area for egg storage and records. We had 200 chickens, Light Sussex and Rhode Island Red. Chicken was on the menu each week so we killed what was for the table and with no fridge in those days they were eaten the same day.

The chickens were free range. There were four large runs and it was a mile to wheel the feeding barrow around. Before milking, the eggs were collected. After milking, the cows were taken down to the field and the milking shed and dairy were scrubbed down. The Herdsman and I had one day off a week but not weekends and if there were any problems, we would stay on. And when it snowed, Ted and I used to sweep from the main road right up to the front door, for any patients that were walking.

I'm not sure why (because milk wasn't of much interest to him) but one of the psychiatrists, Dr Forsyth, had his own cow. She was called Lucette and when she had a calf, both Ted and I were on duty. She had her calf, no bother, and when we'd cleaned up, Ted said: 'Right, we'll both go up and see Dr Forsyth.'

Well he was like a kid: 'Aaah! Why didn't you get me before?' 'Quick delivery,' we said (it wasn't true of course) but as Ted had hoped, he gave us a gin each. While his back was turned, I put mine in a plant but Ted had plenty more and then Dr Forsyth came down to the calving boxes and was very excited. I didn't see that much of Dr Forsyth really but when he came around the yard he was always going to get me in the straw. I could have managed him!

At Christmas we were given five shillings by Dr Brown and on Christmas morning we went to reception and each had a gift from the Christmas tree, which stretched from floor to ceiling. Christmas lunch was held in the maid's sitting room in the basement. The doctor would carve the turkey. We had wine and bonbons and afterwards we could clear the table because we had no supper that night. I didn't know about that at first and wondered why everyone brought a little bag with them. Every January we had a fancy dress dance. One year I did a cancan and got first prize.

Staff were not allowed to use the front drive or front door. Both the front and back doors were locked at 11pm. As I went dancing a lot, I had to use the bell at the side door. Eventually, a grill would be pushed to one side to see who it was, just like a prison. There were many big trees in the grounds and Dr Brown used to hide behind the biggest tree to see who went out early and came in late. At first I thought he was having a piddle but no, he was checking up on us.

Dr Forsyth's father lived at The Priory too. He was always about to die so there were regular parties for him. One time they got the Queen's piper to pipe from the balcony. It was a summer's night and I sat listening, it was beautiful. I think that was his 90th.

Things were changing and when the herd went, Ted and I had to take the cows and calves to Reading to be sold. A hotel was booked for the night for us but we didn't want to leave the cows in case something went wrong. It was heartbreaking to leave them and our dear little calves.

Next, we got hundreds and hundreds of chickens and I helped in the garden when the work was done with the chickens.

I thought The Priory was doing all right but lo and behold it was decided they were going to sell the land. We were devastated. They offered me the job of linen keeper because they'd heard I was handy with my sewing machine. I cried when I left. I was 62. They thought it was time I retired."

Erich Herrmann, Electrician/Butler/Head of Maintenance
Priory Years: 1953 – 1996

It was the winter of '96 when Brian from the maintenance team came into my office and plopped himself down absent-mindedly. I asked why we had no heating. It was still second nature for him to reply, "The German is looking at it now." He didn't realise what he'd said and he trundled off. For a moment I allowed myself the luxury of that cosy feeling again: Erich will fix it. Then I returned to the real world; to a large, meandering old building, every part of which mourned Erich, the guardian of its Gothic eccentricity. He had died on the 30th August that year.

Erich came to England as a German refugee after the war to make a new life for himself. He had to do compulsory work on the Isle of Wight before he was allowed to apply for jobs. His English wasn't too good and he was barely 20 when he saw an advertisement in the paper: *The Priory – London - Electrician*.

London! That meant bright lights. In fact, as Erich was to discover, The Priory had just about the dimmest lights imaginable. He got the job but within days (when he learned that the work of an electrician included carrying out deceased patients), he went to the Engineer to hand in his notice. He was told he'd have to see Dr Brown about that. Dr Brown did his best to persuade him to stay but Erich said it wasn't his scene to work in the dark ages. Then the doctor surprised him, 'Would you consider becoming my butler?' Erich had only the vaguest idea of a butler's duties but the promise of a 5/- a week pay rise swung it. He was measured up for a black suit at a 50-shilling tailor in Putney but refused to go along with the doctor's whim that he should wear a bowler hat.

Many years later, when I occasionally looked in on Erich and the lads early in the morning, they would be in their basement hideout. If Erich was holding the floor, I was in for a treat. Mind you, some mornings he was intent upon extolling the virtues of his trumpeter hero, Harry James, and it was then that Brian would be wearing his Walkman, head deep in *The Mirror*, and John would be in a trance. At other times Erich would entertain with tales of The Priory past. These stories intrigued me because I knew some of the players and because they offered an enticing glimpse into the psychiatry of yesteryear.

It could be said that when Erich was good he was very very good. And when he was bad he was horrid. Particularly in earlier days he was irascible and stubborn at times. If he didn't respect one of our (many) Hospital Directors, he would shape paper airplanes and fly them during management meetings. I would be transfixed, half wondering how he *dared* and half wanting to fly my own plane.

He had a great love of music, particularly jazz. My best-loved musical story was from the Fifties, when he was working in his basement office one day. He had jazz playing on the radio when a figure suddenly appeared in the doorway. Erich immediately realised that this was a patient, who had somehow strayed to the bowels of the building. 'Do you like this sort of music?' the man asked. 'Oh, I love it', Erich replied. 'I have an orchestra you know,' continued the man (*here we go*, thought Erich, *delusions of grandeur*). 'Really? How marvellous', he enthused kindly. Next day the man appeared again, flourishing the gift of a record. Erich was shame-faced to see that he was indeed a famous bandleader.

Another day Erich was doing his rounds of the building and was surprised by a drip then steady flow of liquid, as he walked under a balcony. Looking up, he saw a patient in some disarray. 'What are you doing?' Erich cried. 'I'm piddling on your head!' was the riposte.

Chairman and Chief Executive John Hughes had this to say about Erich:

> "Erich was the only person who knew every wire and pipe in the old rambling building. We had no trade unions, but Erich was the de facto shop steward. He said exactly what he thought and had a socialist's chip on his shoulder regarding management – a straightforward, honest troublemaker for me. After three years or so, one morning I got out of my car and greeted Erich. I knew I'd finally gained his confidence when he turned to give me a small 'Heil, Hitler' salute.
>
> In 1983 we were building Hayes Grove Priory in southeast London (which, incidentally, was the first new private psychiatric hospital opened in Britain since 1920). The job foreman was an old-fashioned London builder who'd fought the Germans and he enjoyed winding Erich up. One day the landscapers unearthed an unexploded German incendiary bomb – an evil looking thing about 24" long. The cockney foreman brought Erich over to see it, and said, "Here's this bomb. It's yours. What are you going to do about it?" Erich, pointing at the bomb, replied, "Vell, it's obvious. It's no gut! I vill take the serial number and report the man who made it!"

Back at The Roehampton Priory, here's a final titbit about Erich. It is just hearsay, and I have wrestled with whether to include it, but I find it ingenious and endearing. It has been said that Erich used to listen in and tape what was going on in board meetings. For these meetings, the chapel became the 'board room' and Erich was in charge of the preparations beforehand. I'm told that he used to feed a microphone from the basement up through a hole in the skirting board within the chapel. He set up a tape recorder in the loo in the basement [the loo is no longer there] and during board meetings he would turn the recorder on. I understand that the cover of the hole for the mike is still there. My source told me: 'There wasn't a lot Erich didn't know. There were shareholders at one time and he was one of the few people given shares. He always knew when to buy and sell!' Is it true? Who knows?

Towards the end of his working life, Erich took to waving a retirement magazine at me, as a tease about his impending departure. When he succumbed to pancreatic cancer instead, it was terribly upsetting for us all.

Before we knew that he was terminally ill, I had told Erich that I wanted to organise a Desert Island Discs-type farewell, with my friend Sheila interviewing him about his Priory life. Once he realised I was serious, that the Kellys would host the event and that all I wanted him to do was choose his records, Erich set about his selections with gusto. But as the reports from his wife worsened, it looked as though he wouldn't make it. Yet he rallied for the occasion and his colleagues watched and listened as he reminisced about his 43 years as electrician come butler come head of maintenance, between playing his beloved jazz records.

His final choice - trumpeter Harry James playing *You Made Me Love You* - was Erich's way of conveying his affection for his Priory colleagues.

Doris Day, Domestic help to Tea Lady
Priory Years: 1953 – 1997

> At the time of this interview in 1991, Doris was 67 and still an integral part of The Priory after 38 years. She was working in the Consultants' area, where she supplied humour and honesty along with tea and biscuits. If her kitchen door was closed it was probably because someone was benefiting from some cheerful and practical counselling. Doris was often referred to as "the psychiatrist's psychiatrist."

"I first came to The Priory in April 1953. I didn't like being on my own, with my husband Henry at work and the kids at school; Valerie was 6 and Billy, 5. Henry had a friend at The Priory who said why didn't I go up there and help out? Not for money but just to spend time. Henry wasn't keen about me being there at first and I didn't tell him little incidents that went on, in case he objected even more.

The patients were elderly, there were no youngsters. I suppose that's why I felt so young; it was the first time I'd been out in the world. I had done one job when I left school, as a Saturday girl, cashier and bookkeeping, but nothing else so I didn't know what to expect from jobs really.

The lady who trained me, Florence Watts, became a good friend. She had been there as a cleaner for a long time and she used to make me laugh. When she first saw me she said, 'What are you doing here?' I said 'I've come to work.' She said 'You're only a bit of a kid.' I said 'I'll have you know I've got two children.' I was cross!

Anyway, a broom was shoved in my hand and I was told that I'd get two shillings an hour and free lunches. I agreed. The corridor I worked on had 15 male patients and all day long you heard the clanking of keys in locks. Before a doctor's visit there was plenty of spit and polish. We certainly knew when Dr Sargant was expected. He was tall, a real gent, and I felt quite important when he walked by! And Dr Flood was the Medical Director then, an extremely nice man with a lovely family. There was a lot of fun about him.

I worked in the area where it was all going on. I wasn't up where the better patients were. You had to keep on the corridor where you worked. You weren't allowed to wander where you wanted in The Priory.

Maintaining The Fabric

We were allowed to get what we needed from stores, and then back to our particular area. We all had our own key and had to hang it up every night before we left; they were checked every night so if you hadn't left yours you were in dead trouble. Every patient was locked in. So to get into a room to clean it you had all these different keys. Male nurses in white overalls were there – you were never left alone with patients. There was an unwritten rule that every lady there would have a sort of guardian who would keep a watch out for you. I had a very nice chap and we were friends right until a few years ago when he died.

In the 1950s some of the rooms were like padded cells. The mattresses were bare and the toilet was a pot in the corner. I had to be a jack of all trades and even fed the patients in the padded cells. You did this by opening the peepholes of their rooms and flicking the food through. I was given a plate of food, fish perhaps, or it could be potato or lumps of meat, and I would feed them through this little hole. The food would fall on the floor and they'd eat it. If you gave it to them on a plate they'd smack it back at you.

They used to lie on bare mattresses because if you gave them sheets they'd tear them up. I must have been ever so lonely to work there but I suppose it all had a horrid fascination.

Once or twice a day the men were escorted outside for some air. I used to watch as they silently shuffled round and round an exercise area, clutching the waists of their trousers. I was told that their belts were usually removed for security reasons. From my point of view, it meant they couldn't chase me because their trousers would fall down. I felt really sorry for them. I don't think some of them could speak; they were in a state of shock from the war.

One day, when a very famous patient ran off down the drive, I was asked to go after her on my bicycle. I peddled along furiously, thinking *Crikey! What an honour!* When I caught up with her, I said in my best voice, 'Excuse me. They want you to go back.' A couple of sharp words told me where to go, and as the nurses had arrived, I went.

There was a lot of land at The Priory then, orchards too, and a few of us used to go scrumping. We came back from the orchard one day with loads of apples in our aprons. We saw a doctor walking towards us so we started to run and all these apples spilt out onto the ground. He knew we'd nicked them but said we might as well keep them. We never went scrumping again, that frightened us!

In those days, Erich Herrmann was the Butler and wore white gloves. When he wasn't butlering he used to help out with the stores and count how much polish we had. Every room had its own fire with sticks and coal. We had to clean them out every morning and then light them. To light the fire quickly, we used polish because we knew it would make it flare. If he caught us he wouldn't half lead off. The polish came in a great big drum and we had our own little tins for him to fill up. He'd go mad if we wanted more polish than he thought we needed. He was a hard man!

My boss was the chief male nurse, Mr Smith, who was in charge of the domestics. To clean the corridors we had a great big heavy bumper. There was no carpet; it was all to be polished. But we were happy, and even used to have a laugh with the patients sometimes.

They used to say 'If you can get on the right side of Doris you'll stay at The Priory and be happy.' I'm going to sue them for definition of character! [Doris was famous for her malapropisms].

Nowadays I take in tea, coffee or lunch when there are board meetings. People say 'Doris must know a thing or two from those meetings,' but I've got real cloth ears. Same as the Monday doctor's lunches, I would never ever repeat what I hear. People ask me why I still come to work here and I explain that having lost my dear Henry I need to keep with my friends.

About 17 years ago, when I was walking through one of the lounges, I was stopped by a patient: 'How long have you been here?' he demanded. 'Oh, more than 20 years now' I replied. 'Good Lord!' he cried, 'Haven't they got you better yet?'"

Clara Guagueta, Cleaner
Priory Years: 1972 - 2006

> Clara remains passionate about The Priory but is even more passionate about her new life with boyfriend David.

"I was born in Bogota, Colombia. I loved being with my family but a friend said I should think about going to England. After university I had worked as a Design Assistant at Lafayette so I had money in the bank to get a ticket.

I thought about it so much that one day I talked to my family. They were very upset because they wanted us all to be together. But one day a letter came from an English family inviting me to go to England to look after their children, to be an *au pair*. My father said: 'Go.' I was twenty.

Later, somebody told me that a place called The Priory needed people. So I got to thinking about that because by then I had done my two years as an *au pair*. I went for an interview with Mr Moore and Gloria Murphy. They were very welcoming but said I needed a permit before I could work there. They thought it could take six months or a year.

Every month my heart went pitter-patter and after six months Mr Moore called me to the office. He said 'Welcome to The Priory Hospital. You have your work permit!' I was given a little room in the nurses' home. The money wasn't much but there was accommodation. I was impressed with The Priory. It was old-fashioned, elegant, and full of old people.

Maintaining The Fabric

When the Americans came to take over the hospital, things changed for the better. There were new managers and Dr Kelly was the Medical Director; this doctor he is very human.

The areas I liked working in most were the doctors' offices and Galsworthy Lodge, the alcohol unit. I loved working at the Lodge. My father was an alcoholic so when I told my mother I was working there she said, 'You must really love them because of your experience with your father.' So when I had the opportunity to speak to them, I did. The Manager, Christina Ball said, 'Why do the patients talk to you so much?!' She didn't really mind and she knew about my father. Christina and I were like sisters, I loved her.

The staff at the alcohol unit were very special people with such good hearts. I met lots of important people there but they smoked such a lot – ashtrays piled so high.

I liked very much Eric Clapton [the famous rock star] when he came to help patients. He is a simple man, lovely to talk to. Some of the patients were snobs and didn't want to talk to me but Eric was very nice. I have very good memories of him and of Gazza.

I worked at Galsworthy Lodge for about 15 years. When I retired, I was working with the bulimic girls at their new unit. That wasn't the best of times. They were so young and it made me so sad, but I tried to support them.

I didn't make any really good friends at The Priory, not because I didn't like the people but because I was working in the evenings. I remember one evening the Housekeeper was walking past the bus stop where I was standing. She stopped and said: 'You're always at the bus stop at this time. Where are you going?' I said 'Oh, I do babysitting for one of my friends.' But what I was really doing was working at the Ritz or the Dorchester Hotel. Doing this was the only way I could afford to go home to Colombia regularly. I kept that secret for 20 years. When the Housekeeper at the Dorchester called me at The Priory, I pleaded, *'Please don't call me at the hospital. Call me on my mobile: I'm not allowed to have two jobs.'*

It was a strange life because during the day in the hospital everyone was sad, they were struggling with bad times, life was hard. But in the evening at the Dorchester, everyone was happy, driving their Bentleys, wearing their fabulous clothes. They were very rich people and gave me tips: £200, £300. And at Christmas I had plenty of envelopes from the guests, with £300 or £400 cash in my Christmas card. One time I had nearly £1,000 in tips. I met Tom Cruise and Nicole Kidman. And Joan Collins, with plenty of wigs – fantastic lady!

So in the evenings I put on my makeup, made sure my uniform was crisp and clean. I would do my manicure and go into the Dorchester with the red nails. One time I was in the corridor when I met my Housekeeper and she said 'Clara! Why are your nails red? You're not allowed to have these. You must take them off.'

And I would have my hair beautifully done and all the other cleaners there would talk about me. I looked very nice in my uniform. It's important to look like a nice girl when you walk into the rooms.

At the Dorchester I had good days and bad days. It was a very hard job. It was only me in the evenings to do 40 rooms. I would get back to The Priory at about 1am, throw my clothes on the floor and collapse into bed.

To keep going in the evenings, I had Coca Cola and a sandwich. In the morning, I had Coca Cola: I was addicted to Coca Cola! When I went to my dentist in Colombia, she said 'What has happened to your teeth? You finish with Coca Cola or you ruin your teeth.'

I met my partner David in Windsor nearly 20 years ago. He was in the museum taking photographs and I was also taking photographs. He was looking at me and we laughed. We started talking and he said 'Would you like to have a coffee?' 'Yes please!' He asked where I lived and I said in London. I gave him my telephone number and he called me after one month. Such a long time! He said he'd been busy. I said I worked very hard too but I would be having a weekend off and so we met in Windsor again. He invited me for lunch and when we parted he gave me a box of chocolates with a lovely card and sweet words, saying he hoped he could see me again soon. I was very happy! I would see David at weekends and he took me to so many places that I now know England better than Colombia.

We have lived together since I retired from The Priory. David is a photographer and we do lots of weddings – David takes the couple and I take the guests. I am very content with life after The Priory."

> See more from Clara in the chapter *Princess Diana and The Priory*.

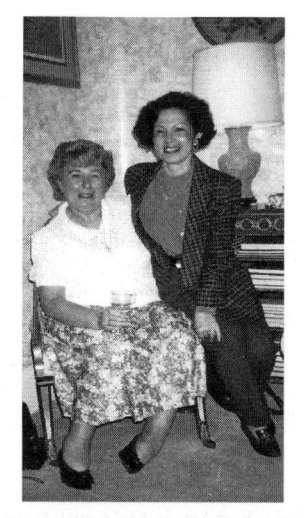

Clara (right) with Doris Day, 1991

Maintaining The Fabric

Robert (Bobby) Smith, Kitchen Porter/Security Officer
Priory Years: 1980 – ongoing

"I started working here at the age of 16, in August 1980. I was in the catering department for 14 months, washing up, a kitchen porter. The building was in bad shape when I started, no doubt about it. I thought, *I'm not going to last a week here*. In the kitchen when it used to rain it was like a shower. We're sitting there washing our hair! There was no need to wash the floor because the rain did it.

Then they fixed the roof and they put a new fan in but it didn't work. And one day we were walking around the kitchen naked. Well, shorts and flip-flops. We had a Spanish chef, Pepe. I loved him and his Spanish singing, and he talked to himself a lot. He was crying, 'Mama Mia Mama Mia, it's a-hotter than a-Spain!' We used to sit in the freezer for a couple of hours to cool down! Without the Americans coming I don't know what would have happened to the place.

I became a housekeeping porter 14 months later. It was less hours, 8am to 4pm, and Saturdays and Sundays if I wanted them. I also cleaned carpets, did the rubbish, cleaned windows - did the post, the papers...

When a patient arrived, Reception staff bleeped me to say that a certain patient was going to a certain room, and while the Admissions Department was sorting the paperwork out, I'd take the luggage to the room. I've actually carried a few patients to their rooms but I'm not sure they were grateful.

We've had some funny requests. Erich said one day, 'Go out the front and put a double white sheet on the lawn.' I told him he was winding me up. He said 'I'm not.' And when I went out, there was a helicopter flying around.

One Saturday morning, I was arriving at work and walking up the front drive when a woman ran across the grass. She was stark naked. I thought I was hallucinating because I'd been to a party the night before and was feeling pretty topsy-turvy. I went in and said to Jill, the receptionist, 'Have a look out there. Can you see a naked woman running around the garden?' She said I was right. I was quite relieved. A nurse went out to fetch her: big girl.

I've chatted with some fantastic people - Eric Clapton, Kate Moss, Gazza. Eric Clapton gave us tickets for a concert at the Albert Hall. In the Royal Box!

When the Chief Executive, John Hughes, first came over from America, he lived at Priory Lodge. I was working one Sunday morning and walked down Priory Lane on my way home and saw him picking plums off his tree. He was struggling so I went to him and said, 'Mr Hughes, I'll help you. I'll climb up the tree and get the top plums for you.'

So I was at the top of this tree, the wind was blowing, the tree was rocking and I was sweating and shitting myself. I got just the plums he wanted, and he said,

'Come in the house, I'll give you something.' I thought, *I'm in here, it'll be a fiver.*

He came out with a whisky glass full of crushed plums! A load of crushed plums! I walked down the road thinking *You bastard! I risk my life and get crushed plums in a whisky glass!* I decided to keep them and show Erich, and left them in the fridge. About a week later, Mr Hughes asked for his whisky glass back. It's a good job I hadn't thrown it away!

I was totally shocked to be employee of the year in 1990, and quite chuffed. There were a couple of people who didn't appreciate it but I think 90% did. It gave me more responsibility somehow, something to live up to.

I have thought *I've had enough of this* a few times over the years, and I've been offered a couple of jobs. But there's something about this place that keeps me here. Of course there's life after The Priory. It would take you down if you couldn't think there was. And you've got to have a life outside these doors. You've got to set yourself new goals. Erich always said, 'If you can work at The Priory, you can work anywhere.'"

A final anecdote from Bobby:

Sole Searching

"I remember one incident many years ago when the senior nurse Danny Appadoo worked on Upper Court. There was a patient acting violently in the back corridor of Wood Wing and eventually we managed to get him on the ground. One of the first things you have to do is take their shoes off so that they can't kick you as well as everything else. Danny was trying to take the patient's shoes off but he wasn't taking his off, he was taking mine off. So in the middle of all the confusion I was trying to tell Danny 'That's my shoes. Hey, that's me!' But he wouldn't listen. Luckily, the patient started laughing his head off and went straight to his room!"

John Whear, Carpenter & Brian Suter, Gardener
Their combined Priory years spanned 1975 - 2007

John the carpenter was a quiet and cuddly kind of guy, who kept his own counsel. He was bright, loyal, lugubrious, bearded and solid. He took life seriously yet was witty in a deadpan sort of way. He was devoted to his dogs, who went everywhere with him. Very sadly, he died in 2007 while still working at the Marchwood Priory.

As for Brian, when he wasn't in the garden he used to cruise the building, slapping a paintbrush around, changing bulbs and unblocking toilets. Meanwhile, he would soak up information like a sponge and was therefore very well-informed.

When we got together at my flat, John Whear had been with the company for 24 years. By then, however, he was working at Marchwood Priory in Southampton. Brian joined the Roehampton Priory in 1986 and left in 2004. The two of them had many anecdotes and here, in no particular order, are some of them.

"John: I was self-employed and a friend, Dave the carpet man, said 'Are you interested in doing a bit of work up at The Priory?' I said 'What is it?' He said 'I don't know but go and see a bloke called Erich Herrmann and he'll tell you what it is'. That was 1975.

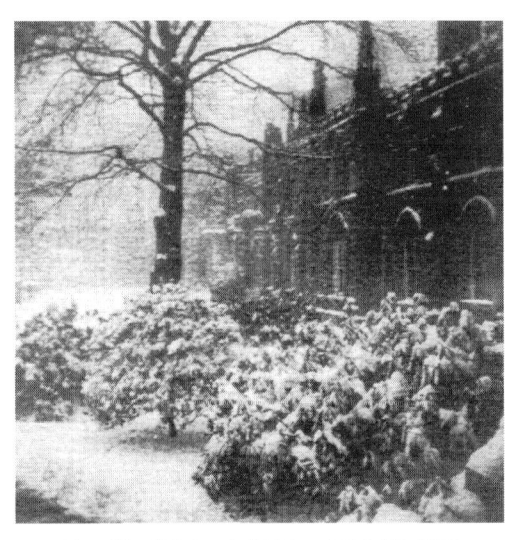

How The Priory would have looked to John

I realised I'd been there once before, when I was an apprentice. That was about 1968 when we had the bad winter and there was snow on the ground for three weeks. I was on my way home from night school and it was very foggy. I was on my push bike and a car tooted from behind. I stopped and a man said 'Do you know where The Priory is?' I said no. 'Do you know where Roehampton is?' 'Oh yes, I know Roehampton.' 'Could you show me how to get there?' So I took him all the way to Roehampton – me on my push bike and him in his Jag.

When we found it we went up the drive, through a ramshackle old wooden gate. I hung around outside while he went in and picked up his relative. I knew it was some sort of hospital. He must have been about an hour. It was freezing cold and pitch black. Then he wanted me to take him back to Knightsbridge! I said 'I'll take you back as far as Kensington, and from there it's a straight road.'

I got him to Kensington and he gave me a fiver, which was a lot of money then.

But I ended up with great big chilblains and I didn't get to bed until three in the morning because I still had to cycle all the way back to Barnes. I was stupid in those days.

So I went to do this job and met Erich. He'd seen the ceiling in the cafeteria at Queen Mary's Hospital and wanted it in the staff canteen. It was just slats of wood at a 45 degree angle across the ceiling, with a bit of space above. I said 'Alright, you supply the materials, I'll supply the labour.'

When I had finished, he said, 'Are you interested in coming to work for us?' I said 'What's the money?' He mentioned some sort of pittance. I said 'Not interested.' Another job at The Priory came up and I did that and the offer was made again and the money went up a little bit. Four or five times later, I said 'What are you offering this week?' It wasn't as much as I was earning but I was getting really cheesed off with being self-employed.

It wasn't until 15 years later that Erich told me why he had wanted me so badly. It was to get a fire certificate for the place. It was in really bad condition, and I spent the best part of 12 years making fire doors. Of course as soon as we got anywhere near the specifications (which might take 18 months to achieve) a new set of regulations came in so we had to get on with that. We eventually got the certificate in about 1986.

But in 1975 the place was like a Victorian workhouse: horrible. The corridors were lit every thirty feet by fluorescent tubes. There were still fireplaces in all the rooms, ceilings with 40 watt bulbs in the middle of the rooms, no shades. There were single rooms but no en-suite bathrooms. There were carpet squares in the middle of the room and floorboards painted black around them.

We had a lot of old people, mostly long stay patients. There was a good track record for keeping people alive, no doubt about it. They celebrated one old girl's birthday when she was 105 years old.

That's why they weren't making any money. The relatives set up trust funds for the patients, and of course fees went up but they'd signed contracts. They were probably paying £200 a month to keep the patient there and it would actually be costing the hospital £300 or £400, bare minimum.

The Priory was owned by a family and Dr John Flood was the head doctor and had a lot of shares in the place as well. Then the family wanted to sell up and, according to Erich, Dr Flood was in dire straits – he couldn't raise the money. He was about £75,000 short and the deadline was that day. And a John Marsh happened to be there as a patient. He saw Dr Flood and said, 'You look all done. You should be in here rather than me.' John Flood told him what the problem was, and he got his cheque book out and wrote a £75,000 cheque; went into the board room and said 'Right, I think that makes me Chairman.' So that was when Mr Marsh took over.

He used to turn up in his 7 litre Mercedes, with his chauffeur. He would get there at 5 o'clock in the morning, catch all the night staff sleeping, go round and turn all the fridges down, turn all the lights off and generally try to save a few pennies.

It was later that Dr Flood got Mr Vinacour [Administrator] to go over to the States to get Community Psychiatric Centers (CPC) interested. Old man Conte [founder of CPC] came to look at the place and when they arrived at Heathrow, Erich was duly sent to pick them up. He gave them the royal tour, through Richmond Park and down Priory Lane. When they came down the drive and first caught a glimpse of the building Mrs. Conte said: 'Oh My God, look at this. It's just like Disneyland. We've got to have it.' So basically it was signed and sealed there and then. That was the start of CPC in this country.

Brian: I joined in June 1986, having seen an ad at the job centre for a gardener with qualifications. My interview was with Peter Gwatkin on the front lawn. The first thing he said was 'We're going to try contractors actually. We'll pay your expenses for coming, obviously. But can you help us out for a couple of days in the garden? We've got a seminar coming up.' I didn't know what a seminar was but said ok. He said 'The man you've got to see is German, and he's on holiday at the moment. His name's Erich, come in Monday morning and he'll find you some tools.' I turned up 9 o'clock on Monday morning, saw Erich, got the tools. Tuesday afternoon, he came out and offered me a position. And I've been there 12½ years.

On my first day, I didn't know anything except that there were very well-to-do psychiatric patients about. This gentleman came across the lawn and I thought *Hello, here comes one of them*. He said 'How do you do, I'm John Hughes, the Chief Executive, welcome to the company.' I did wonder, I must admit.

John: During the summer you couldn't get Brian out of the garden, but during the cold weather he used to creep in.

Brian: What people don't realise is that in gardening you have to tackle virtually every trade – from bricklaying to a bit of electrics to a bit of plumbing – unfortunately Erich found out that I could do these things.

John: I remember a patient who used to call me 'Jesus', because of my beard. One day she was out on the front lawn, having this thing about loving everyone. She came across the lawn, put her arms around me in a bear hug and was telling me that she loved me, just as twenty patients on a Priory walk were going across the lawn! I said 'Put me down!' She used to sunbathe naked in the secure garden.

It's funny you know, in the 20 odd years I worked at The Priory I never saw a patient in the nude, not once. I was always in the wrong place at the wrong time. The nearest I got to it was on a corridor once when I opened a door. There was a patient on the floor with her nightdress on, shouting at the top of her voice: 'I am a fish! I am a fish!' while a couple of nurses tried to stop her swimming down the corridor.

Two more stories then we must go. When John Flood first arrived, he had come out of the army. He was the psychiatrist who looked after people when they came back from Japanese prison camps. He wanted to go into private practice so came to The Priory as a junior doctor.

The head male nurse was showing him through the gents side and Dr Flood saw a patient with a toothbrush on the end of a piece of string. He was pulling this bit of string along behind him with the toothbrush on the end. So John Flood thought, *he thinks it's a dog*. He spoke to him: 'That's a lovely dog you've got there.' The patient looked at him and said 'That's not a dog. It's a toothbrush.' John Flood said 'Ah!' Two or three yards further on he heard the patient say, 'That fooled him Fido!'

I miss The Priory terribly. I'd love to get back there."

Their last anecdote:

Moses in the Mortuary
"We had a mortuary in earlier days because most of our clients were old people and they used to kick the bucket on a fairly regular basis. In fact the maintenance staff used to have the job of carrying them to the mortuary and we used to get a bottle of Guinness each to do it.

Moses was an Afro-Caribbean plumber. Well, he called himself a plumber. Anyway, the mortuary wasn't being used by the time he worked there and we had to shift some furniture. The only place we could store it was the old mortuary. Moses had never been there before and Steve and Kevin thought they'd have a bit of a laugh.

Moses was carrying one end of a bit of furniture and he saw the big slab and the wooden block for the head and he said 'What's this?' Steve said 'This is the mortuary. It's where they lay them out before the undertaker comes to collect them.' That really flustered Moses.

Next day, we had to carry more furniture in there but first of all, Steve got this bed sheet and a cardboard label, took his shoes and socks off, tied the label on his toe, lay down on the slab and covered himself up with the sheet. Moses comes in and his eyes widen. Suddenly this corpse sits up and Moses runs out screaming. We didn't see him for three days, when he handed his notice in!"

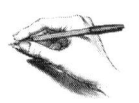

The reunion with my son was planned for the 2nd July 1991, at the agency, and in the presence of the social worker, Rose. I had mixed feelings about this; it seemed such a private thing, surely Rose would be in the way? But she said it was helpful to have someone else present, someone used to reunions and who could mediate when necessary.

The arrangements were precise: Robert would arrive at noon and I would arrive 15 minutes later. This was to save us from meeting without ceremony on the doorstep. All morning I panicked. I was abrupt when people phoned to wish me luck, sure that I wasn't the sort of mother Robert would want, and convinced that I would dreamily crash the car. A friend had actually offered to be our driver for the day. He would wear a chauffeur's cap, he said, and be terribly discreet and professional. I didn't believe this and knew he would spend all his time looking in the rear view mirror to see how we were getting along. Anyway, it would have created a completely false impression as to my financial situation. And above all, I wanted to be alone with my thoughts on the way to our reunion and on the way home again.

Anyone watching me teeter from the car to the agency would have thought me drunk, rheumatic, or both. My knees were giving way, heart pounding and face burning.

Rose was at the door. "Robert has arrived," she smiled. "Are you ready to see him, or...?" "Or" I said, making for the loo. When I emerged, she led me up the fateful stairs and into the room where my son was waiting.

This was it: the moment I had waited for. Would we shake hands, embrace, weep? Would we collapse in a heap? We did none of these things. We could barely look at each other, apart from brief sideways glances. Giggling self-consciously, we sat gingerly on the sofa and stared fixedly at Rose (so much for thinking she would be in the way).

We talked about how we were feeling, about the information Robert had *gathered over the years and about how we might spend the day. An hour later Rose released us upon the world: "Don't spend too long together" she warned. "You will be emotionally exhausted."*

We had lunch at one of my favourite pubs in Richmond, followed by a long walk beside the river. I showed Robert some photos of himself as a baby and we wept and hugged and wept some more. By the time I dropped him back at the agency to collect his own car, I knew that Rose had been right, we were emotionally exhausted.

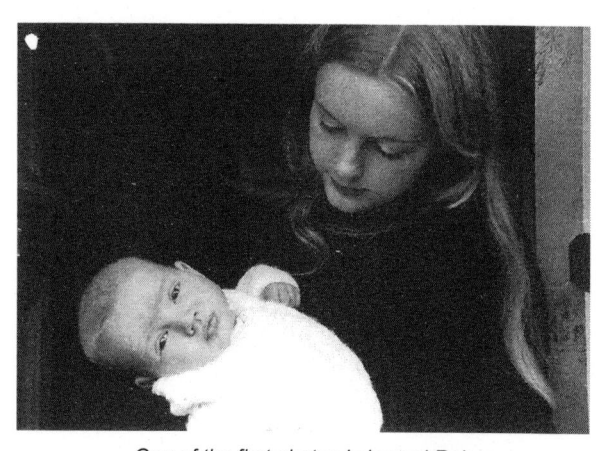

One of the first photos I showed Rob

This is how Rob described the day afterwards:

> After smoking 63 packets of cigarettes, and inevitably losing my way in London, I reach the agency. 15 minutes late – typical – what if I bump into her on the stairs – what am I going to say?
>
> I meet Rose Wallace and head for the security of her office and a cup of coffee which I half drink, half spill on the carpet. I am feeling anxious. No, I'm not, I'm bloody panicking.
>
> The next 17 minutes are the longest of my life. Do I look alright? Oh no, my trousers are creased. I'm done for – no ironing board here and if there were, did I have time to whip my trousers off and iron them? The polo mint helped but I was blissfully unaware that it was obvious to any sensitive non-smoker that I was a smoker. Damn - and to think I didn't know how to tell her!
>
> Then we're told that she's arrived. Rose goes to get her. What on earth are they doing down there? I'm sure the stairs weren't as long as all that.
>
> In she breezes, my roots, my blood. The faceless figure I had

dreamt about during my childhood was standing in front of me, smiling. 'Very nice' I waffled. What else could I say? My mind went to pieces, exploding in a billion different directions at once.

We sat down. I was in a state of major emotional contradictions, being happy and worried that I'd portray myself acceptably. I wanted her to like me, to be proud of me, and God did I need a cigarette.

The rest of the day was a hazy dream. It went well, walking, talking and not eating much. I was happy and I liked my new found Mum.

So, after an embarrassed and longed-for short cuddle, I drove home on air and reflected on the day. 'A dream come true' was my conclusion."

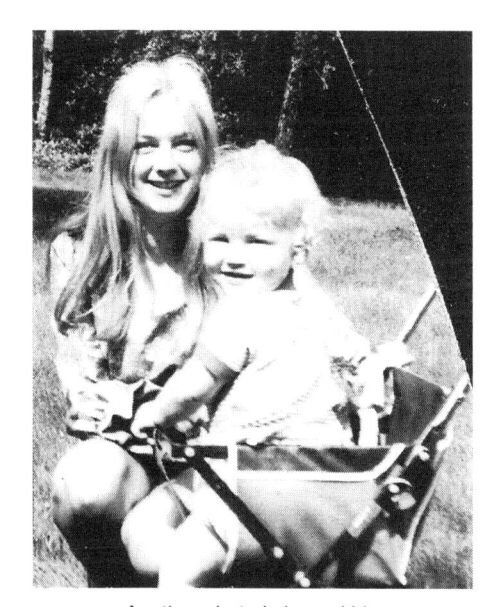

Another photo I showed him

7
Dispensing Care

Virginia Jervis, Pharmacist
Priory Years: 1988 - 2006

"When I started at The Priory as a locum, the sun was shining and I rounded the corner to this wedding cake of a building. People were spilling out over the front lawn and I was warmly greeted by the Director of Nursing, Betty Naudeer, on the main steps. 'Would you like to go and help yourself from the buffet table in the Blue Room?' No, it wasn't all to greet me; it was one of The Priory's famous seminar days, with a sumptuous spread. What a start! I'm sure I was introduced to loads of people but it was all a bit overwhelming. The pharmacy (then in the basement), brought me back to earth with a bump.

The previous Pharmacist only had time – two mornings a week – to do a basic purchasing role. Much of the ordering and preparation of TTO's (medication 'to take out') was done by the nursing staff. But as my hours increased, I gradually extended my role and insisted that the pharmacy should come out of the basement into a more prominent position within the hospital.

When appropriate, I gave one-to-one counselling to patients, held medication awareness groups, and was given the freedom to introduce other new aspects. Mainly, this was down to working faster to generate the time for these extras but I did eventually manage to get some part-time help.

It was quite a while before I attended my first case conference. I had been told by the nursing staff that you had to wait to be invited to attend. Initially, I was in awe of those meetings; partly because of my inexperience and partly because of their formality.

The format was very much like a clinical examination for the trainee doctors. They had to present the case and make the differential diagnosis. Each of the consultants was then asked to comment and to make suggestions for treatment and on-going therapy. I learnt a tremendous amount from those sessions. Later, as I gained the confidence of the consultants, I was invited to make comments too.

Dr Kelly was a tremendous Medical Director. He was passionate about the job and that permeated through the hospital. In a quiet, caring and efficient way (thanks also to Dorothy's organisational skills) he set, and maintained, very high standards. Of course he was a great listener and made it very easy for me to talk things through if I had concerns about, for example, prescribing practice.

I never really felt threatened by patients, although I had to duck a couple of times when a 'missile' flew through the air! Over the years, some very sick people were admitted and they were challenging both in their behaviour and in their pharmaceutical requirements. For example, Dr Kelly's overseas obsessive patients needed lengthy amounts of time.

Pharmacy can be a very remote profession unless you get involved. By that I mean that patients can merely be a name on a prescription that you dispense, unless you get to know the person behind the name. Visiting the wards, especially first thing in the morning, meant that I kept my finger on the pulse. I was able to quickly pick up if I needed to be concerned about a new patient's medication chart or if I needed to order a medication not generally stocked. Talking on a one-to-one basis with patients was often reassuring for them but also rewarding for me.

In later years, I was able to guide some of the junior nursing staff on such things as medication administration techniques or essential monitoring – skills that are no longer taught in nursing school. I'm proud to say that the various inspections by pharmaceutical bodies, pharmacy inspectors etc. all passed with flying colours in my department.

If I were to analyse what made Priory staff love working there, I'd say that you were made to feel valuable; you were a vital cog in the working wheel; people were prepared to help each other for the good of the whole and patients appreciated (mainly!) what was done for them.

At times, though, it felt that things were tough and we started the Fun Committee as something to unite all grades of staff. And it did help. We arranged some very memorable occasions, which have been talked about ever since. The committee (non-elected) enjoyed many noisy lunchtimes, arranging forthcoming events.

No one moment could sum up the complexity of The Priory but there are times that stick in the mind, such as a patient crying on my shoulder with thanks a couple of weeks after I had spent 3 hours trying to explain that her antidepressant medication would not cause addiction; shielding a patient from jumping onto the lines at Barnes Station, and painting Dr Shur's toenails for *Blind Date*!

I had been introduced to Sheila Coyle during my first week at The Priory in January 1982, at a Treatment of Depression seminar. She was the widow of Peter Coyle, who had run the Galsworthy House alcohol unit on Kingston Hill. John Hughes talks about Peter within the chapter An American Rocks

Roehampton. Peter had died in December '81, a month earlier.

A few days after the seminar, I was opening a window at my flat in Philbeach Gardens, Earls Court, and by golly there was that lady Sheila from the seminar, standing directly opposite. "Hello!" I yelled, "what are you doing here?" She waved and called back: "I've lived here for 23 years!" And so began a wonderful friendship. Sheila was one of the first people to meet my new found son, when we spent a delightful afternoon together.

The thought of meeting my brother Jim and his wife Christine, not to mention their four children, Ruth, Helen, Adrian and Carolyn, threw Rob into a tizzy. We were to have lunch with them in Marlow and that morning while I ate breakfast, Rob paced, sighed, groaned and held his tummy. By the time we reached Marlow we were both apprehensive. He had already received letters from his cousins, welcoming him back to the family. Their sentiments included a statement from the youngest, Carolyn, that if he hadn't found us, she would have hired a private detective to find him!

Within minutes of meeting, our large family gathering had taken over a section of the bar and everyone was talking at once. The cousins hit it off immediately and, as Helen, my second niece, said later "You can tell he's one of the family; it's almost an animal thing. He just smells right." For me, to have my own little family unit was absolute heaven.

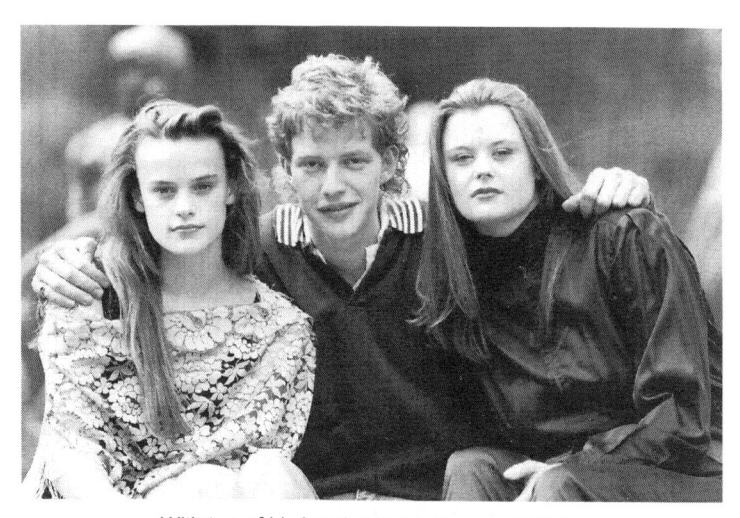

With two of his 'new' cousins, Carolyn & Helen

My sister Susan and her boyfriend John had exchanged letters with Rob too, and came over from America very excited about meeting him.

I also took Rob to meet Dr Kelly. It was a Saturday morning so there were no staff in the Secretariat and most doctors were on the wards. Rob was wary of meeting a psychiatrist and had been fretting about what to wear, so we were both a bit nervous as we approached his office. But when DK made the ludicrous statement that Pink Floyd was his No. 1 group too (surely preposterous), a huge smile came over Rob's face and I sat back gratefully as they chatted away.

"Your mother will have given you some very good, hard-working genes!" was DK's parting shot as we left.

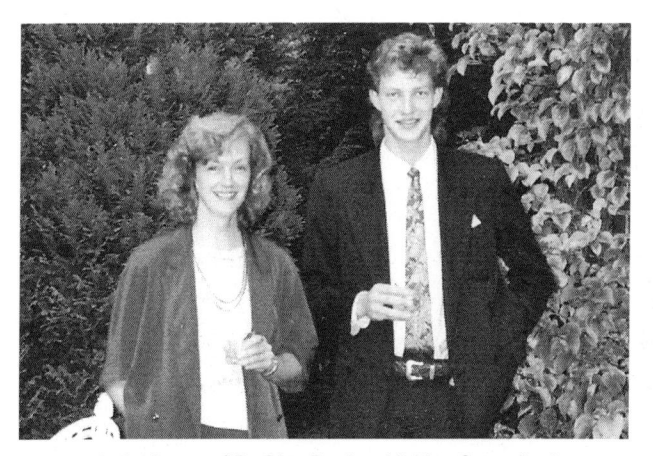

At the home of Dr Glyn Davies, Visiting Consultant

Rob and I wrote to each other frequently. One note from him simply read:

> 'Our Maintenance Man, Chris, said the other day "Christ, look at your ears – no wonder your mother put you up for adoption." So now I know.'

8
Naval Commander Opts For Dry Land

David Wakefield
Priory Years:
Hospital Director 1983 – 1985
Operations Director 1985 – 1988
Managing Director 1988 – 1993
Chairman 1993 - 1996

"I decided to leave the Navy after the Falklands War because I knew that would be my last sea-going appointment and I couldn't really see much point in staying in the Navy if I could never go to sea again. My final appointment was as Commander (Logistics) in HMS Antrim and after that I would just have had desk jobs at the Ministry of Defence and maybe one or two countries abroad. The Navy was getting smaller and it seemed to me, at 35, that if I was going to leave, now was the time to do it. I was wondering what my next career might be and – arrogantly maybe – thought that if I could run a warship I could run a hospital. It's all a question of moulding together a bunch of people of different disciplines to achieve a common end.

Initially, I looked for healthcare jobs in the NHS. But in those days the NHS had no concept of taking in people who already had significant experience elsewhere. They expected you to join as a youngster and be with them for life. So I started looking into the private sector and saw an advertisement that said CPC Private Hospital Management. I applied and was interviewed by John Hughes, the Chairman, at The Priory in October 1982 and was offered the job in the November. I started in January '83 and left the company when it was sold to Mercury Development Capital in June 1996.

I got on well with John and liked the idea of the private sector because there were more resources available to care for patients. The patients were clearly being looked after extremely well and I felt this was something I could identify with; I could share its values and believed I could make a contribution. I felt comfortable and confident.

I also got on extremely well with Desmond Kelly. I liked what he told me about his philosophy and approach to caring for patients and the whole ethos of The Priory. He assured me that since the American company CPC had taken over, things were much better and that money was being invested in The Priory and that refurbishment work was taking place. There seemed to be a real commitment to make it a first class establishment.

I was Hospital Director at The Priory between January 1983 and the summer of 1985, when I became the Operations Director. At that time we had opened two further hospitals: Hayes Grove Priory in Kent and the Woodbourne Clinic in Birmingham.

John Hughes, who had been the first Chairman and Chief Executive of the Group, was asked to go back to America in 1987 but he declined and left the company to set up his own psychiatric services company in the UK. Bob Derenthal, a Senior Vice President in the US, arrived to take over. Bob was there until 1988, at which point he returned to the United States and I became the Managing Director and Desmond Kelly became the Chairman.

In the Navy, everyone knows their place. That isn't to say they're subservient – they're not, they're bright people and they use a lot of initiative in what they do. But it is a hierarchical structure. If you need to give an order, or indeed you're just going about your day-to-day business and you say to somebody I want this, they do it. Because that's the way the Navy is, people are trained to do that. There's a mechanism in the Navy that if they think that what you are asking them to do is not the best way of doing it, there are ways of saying so. And they will; they're not automatons by any means.

At The Priory of course, being a civilian organisation and a medical one at that, a lot of people weren't used to being given instructions of any sort whatsoever. Many people had their own agenda and what I found initially quite surprising and a bit curious was that people were quite rigid about what they would and wouldn't do. On the other hand, they didn't want to take responsibility for anything they regarded as being out of their patch. So it was quite a steep learning curve for me, to find ways of managing people who didn't automatically respond to what I requested of them.

There was no sense of 'Americanism' in The Priory at all. I think John Hughes, maybe deliberately, had not tried to foster that. He was also very busy trying to open up new businesses for CPC and I don't think he spent a huge amount of time pondering the culture of the hospital. He let other people get on with that.

When I joined, John had already found the site at Hayes Grove and that was being built. He used to take me over there and show me what they were doing, discuss the business plan for Hayes and the consultant recruitment programme and clearly wanted to bring me into the decision making process for new hospital development.

John is actually a significant entrepreneur, a very good businessman, and I learned a lot from him and was grateful that he took me into his confidence very early on, both by allowing me to get on with running The Priory with almost no interference but also by sharing his ideas and plans for other developments.

If I were critical, I would say that John didn't mentor me enough in some ways, in as much as I was an ex-Naval Officer. Yes, I'd had a lot of management experience in the ways of the Navy and I had a fair amount of financial experience in running the large budget of a warship. But that's not the same as running a profit and loss account for a business. I think he just assumed I could get on with it and I guess as the monthly results started coming in and the hospital was doing ok, he decided I *could* get on with it.

John was a business role model, certainly, for his acumen, huge energy, and vision, yet I wouldn't say he was a natural leader. But look at him now: he's highly successful and he's done extremely well. And like all good entrepreneurs he's taken his company to the wire more than once but he's got out of it each time with ultimate success.

I had never been to The Priory before I joined the company, although I had heard of it. When you drive through the gateway and start to see the white building through the trees, then turn the corner and there's the big willow tree and that front portico with its arches, you think "Oh my goodness! This is extraordinary!" And that impression continued because by the time I was there, the reception area and the two big rooms either side had been refurbished and were really quite stunning.

Imagine what it was like for a patient! They're told they're going to a psychiatric hospital and see, in effect, a stately home. And not just a stately home in the sense that it's grand and expensive but it gave an air of tranquillity and calm. So I think that if anyone were anxious or agitated and were suddenly surrounded by this wonderful building and its landscaped grounds, it would be difficult to feel anything other than calmed by that. I wish I'd known it when it had all the land, which is now the Dowdeswell Estate. But even so, the land we had at the front was still pretty impressive.

I didn't have a huge amount of contact with patients. In my early days I would go to groups if invited. I would spend nights on the wards. Of course the patients by and large were asleep, but I'd see what was going on. I didn't seek out the patients – I didn't think it was appropriate that I should do so. Sometimes they wanted to talk about some administrative matter, in which case I'd certainly go and see them. I saw more of the long stay patients that we had then. They used to like me to go and talk to them. When I came there were 27 long stay patients, including two men.

My main challenges on a personal basis were to understand the financial expectations of an American company and to manage the tension between making a profit for the company and not in any way skimping on resources for the patients.

Many health care staff didn't understand cost economy, let alone the idea of making a profit. I'm sure it's changed now but in those days, almost by definition, all of our health care staff came from the NHS, where they had a somewhat laissez faire attitude towards using resources.

I used to say 'Look, if you waste money like this, there will be less money for me to put into patient services, or to improving your terms and conditions.' I just tried to balance one against the other so that they could see there was a finite pot of money and if they chucked something away, they couldn't use it for something else.

Inside The Priory

I think there are three key ingredients needed for people to enjoy their work. If the product of your job is attractive; if you feel your company values you and communicates with you, and gives you reasonable terms of service, then generally you've got a winning formula and I think that's what we had at The Priory. Even in the early days, when perhaps the pay and conditions weren't that good, people responded to the fact that they were in an environment where they were valued and patients were getting well, and that's attractive.

There were some real characters amongst the staff. I remember Doris Day the tea lady for her cheerfulness and easy banter with the doctors and with me, particularly when we had our Monday lunch in the chapel. She came into board meetings too and on one occasion, Richard Conte [son of the founder of CPC] discovered she was wearing red bloomers. That became legendary: Doris and her red bloomers.

The nursing sisters, Renée and Camille, I would exchange a few words of French with them when they were on the Lower Court nursing station. They were always pulling my leg slightly about my lifestyle. They liked the sound of the skiing, good food and music; they thought that was all very appropriate and wanted to talk to me about it!

With Erich Herrmann, the Maintenance Manager, I was always very clear about what I wanted from him and his department and he knew that if I said I wanted something done I'd check up on it. Other than that I let him get on with things. Very quickly, he would do anything I wanted him to do and he'd also let me know about the things that were going on. He became a very good conduit for information for the non-clinical departments and sometimes even the clinical. He wasn't a telltale but if he thought there was something that was not going well, he'd tell me. He was a very good colleague. I liked Erich a lot and got on with him extremely well.

The Chef, Aziz, was a bit of a handful although his heart was in the right place. He was somebody who took the cost control measure too much the other way and was forever trying to cut back. He had little concept of working with other people or being a little flexible. If he could do what he wanted to do, he was good. If you wanted him to do something a bit out of the ordinary or asked him to give the nurses a bit more tea this month, he'd say 'I can't do that.'

I found, generally speaking, that Priory doctors, and the ones we worked with in the NHS, were pretty straightforward, which was a welcome surprise. If you had met them outside The Priory you wouldn't have known they were doctors, let alone psychiatrists. Yet in the Navy (which had very few psychiatrists), we always used to call them 'trick-cyclists', because they were often strange people.

I first met Jim Conte [the founder of CPC] and his son Richard when they came over for the opening of Hayes in November '83. One thing about working for an American company, particularly under Jim's regime, was that Jim and his colleagues in America did not see The Priory in the UK as a separate company.

They just thought it was a division of CPC and they'd send me stupid memos telling me to do things which may or may not be fine in America but were quite ridiculous over here. And I had to decide whether to reply to them or drop them in the bin.

We always made good profits and punched above our weight in that regard. In the year or two before The Priory was finally sold, the UK group of, by that time 14 hospitals and some other businesses, was making more money than the American psychiatric division of goodness knows how many hospitals.

In John Hughes' time I had a hand in developing Hayes, but that was a learning curve; a bit more with Birmingham. In 1986 we had three hospitals coming together – Altrincham, Grovelands, and Marchwood. I set up Altrincham and John did Marchwood and Grovelands, although I assisted with those. Then of course he left and after that I did all the further developments – Bristol, Chelmsford, Leeds, Glasgow, the Dialysis Unit in Rotherham, the children's homes, Eden Grove and Harwich...

So in 1988 when I became the MD, I took over the developments of the company. That was hugely satisfying; to acquire a building, get it set up with doctors on board and staff and the first patients in. And again we continued The Priory tradition of getting some very attractive buildings; a lovely hospital down in Bristol; another in Chelmsford. Glasgow was an interesting joint venture with another hospital and Grovelands in North London – a Grade 1 Listed Nash building. It was fantastic to have taken over a building like that - in a sense restoring it for the nation. It was falling into rack and ruin under local authority and NHS ownership.

It was also very satisfying to see people get well, and we had an extremely good record for that. I won't say curing people – that's a difficult term to use in psychiatry, particularly with addictions – but ensuring they left the hospital in a very much better state than when they arrived. Invariably we achieved that and in many cases people left us never to return because they were well.

The Registrar rotations [see *Trail Blazing Academy*] were a wonderful accolade for The Priory. They were a complete first in the private sector. Initially, Desmond would make contact with the appropriate people at Charing Cross, UCL or St George's Medical Schools, and then I would come in to talk about what would be financially possible and about the associated administrative arrangements. We had to make it attractive to them. As long as they could see there was a net inflow of money into the NHS, and that the clinical training and experience on offer at our hospitals was good, they were happy.

As to admissions, anyone coming in to be treated for drugs or alcohol would have me checking who was going to fund it and how. Usually they weren't covered by insurance. They'd give all sorts of reasons why they weren't going to pay a deposit up front and you just had to make a judgement about whether they were good for their money or not. They were the ones who were most likely not to be good for their money. They were also some of the best people at covering it up because if you can be in denial about addiction you can be in denial about all sorts of things.

We would do some research and be quite tough with them or whoever was bringing them in. We'd tell them what the treatment was going to cost and ask how they were going to pay for it. I would say I needed a deposit, references, assurance that they could cover the whole cost. It was no good for any of us if half way through there's no more money because while I would hate to do it, they'd have to go. So I just tried to make the consequences clear.

We did carry the cost of some patients who ran out of money. Sometimes quite genuinely because their insurance cover, say, was for four weeks and the consultant after a while said they were going to need six weeks. If they couldn't pay anything more we'd work as quickly as we could and take the cost.

There were well-known people who took the line 'You know who I am? I can pay,' and come the crunch, they couldn't pay. You'd have to heavy up on them or their agent – sometimes successfully sometimes not. We always carried a degree of bad debt but it was never high. I can't remember the exact percentage but I'd be surprised if it was ever more than 1% of turnover and probably less. When I joined The Priory there were actually quite a lot of bad debts and I was able to improve the first year profits by bringing some of those in, or at least deciding which ones were collectible and which ones were hopeless.

With Middle Eastern Embassies, in some ways the problem was that they probably didn't owe us enough money. Every so often I'd go into town to the embassies and ask to see the Financial Attaché and tell them this is what you owe and it's affecting our cash flow and the credibility of your country. They'd be amazed that I'd even bothered to ask them for money.

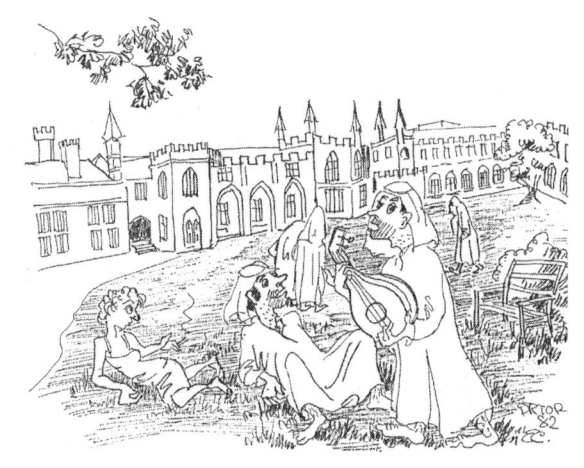

A patient's tongue-in-cheek representation of The Priory in the 1980s

Sometimes they'd shrug and go over to a filing cabinet, open a drawer and pull out Priory letters, each of which had a cheque attached, probably several months old, and say 'Here you are,' and I'd walk away with cheques worth £45,000! To them it was small change and they couldn't see why I was so bothered. And if patients weren't embassy backed, I would want money up front. They'd complain a bit and I'd say 'Come on, I know you can do this, you're an important family, get me a bank transfer', and they did.

Whereas mental illness had perhaps been covered up in the Middle East before, when they discovered they could be treated outside their home country, then the wealthier ones wanted that. Doctors such as Galal Badrawy were bringing patients back and of course once you've brought one patient back the news starts to spread that The Priory in London can help you.

There were a few times when I thought the percentage of Arab patients became too large for comfort, just because it started to change the atmosphere of the hospital. There wasn't much we could do about it. I don't think we ever said no more Arab patients; we just waited until the situation balanced itself, which it did.

They were largely replaced by NHS patients, which was interesting. I think the initial approach came from the NHS to The Priory and it was clearly an opportunity for us. We had the space to do it, felt that we should do it, and gained further credibility for our ability to tackle these patients. We knew full well what would happen. Once any of the London hospitals for whom we were acting as overflow reached that point, they would do as probably anyone would do, which was send us the most difficult patients and keep the easy ones for themselves.

So we did get some very challenging patients. But unlike the NHS, because of the way we were structured, we would start dealing with them straight away. They would see a Registrar on admission, see a Consultant within 24 hours, and a treatment programme would start.

In the earlier days, the NHS wanted them back as soon as they had a spare bed, so we'd just get treatment started and they'd then go back to the general hospitals, which was no good because they might not be seen by anyone for a week. Meanwhile, three days later because the NHS would again have overfill, somebody else would come to us. This rather pointless cycle would continue. So we said 'Look, when you send us a patient, why don't you let us keep them until we've got them to the point where they can be sensibly discharged back to you and if it means you've got a bed empty for a day or two surely that's better than mucking around the patients like this.'

They actually decided that we should keep them until they were ready for a reasonable discharge. And of course they very quickly noticed that many of the patients who came to The Priory were getting better rather more quickly than the ones being treated by the NHS because of the greater intensity of our treatment and because of the environment.

Inside The Priory

I always made it clear to the Hospital Directors that as far as I was concerned each hospital was a separate business. Yes, they had to run their hospital within The Priory ethos and guidelines but they were accountable for the success or failure of their hospital. The overall approach was 'Keep me in the picture. If you're concerned about something, let me know what it is, preferably with an action plan to put it right. Otherwise I won't get in your way.' And that applied to the Roehampton Priory as well as everywhere else. I think The Priory staff perhaps felt a bit vulnerable with Head Office in the grounds, but for the most part we maintained a peaceful separation.

Our partnership with the NHS got the patients numbers up. It was good for our staff to deal with a different type of tricky patient and it was good for our reputation. We felt it would be wrong to have an NHS wing. We just tried to put them into the part of the hospital that was appropriate to their clinical condition. Desmond tells the story of an NHS patient who, during an inspection of the hospital by the local health authority, was asked whether he wanted to leave The Priory. He said: 'What?! Do you think I'm mad?!'

There weren't any bad aspects as such, other than (for me) the disappointing facet that the NHS seemed to have such low expectations of its psychiatric service. In some ways, and I hope that's changed now, they seemed to regard it as a sort of pick up the bits, patch up, keep the lid on type of service rather than really get people sorted out.

Competition meanwhile was increasing. Charter [a main competitor] was quite aggressive and there were others groups coming in to the sector who wanted to take a chunk of it. We were lucky because we had a head start and we had our reputation. My job was to make sure that we remained both the biggest and the best and the hospitals experienced surprisingly few tricky situations or negative publicity.

We had very few suicides. Three, I think, in fourteen years, which was remarkable, given the nature of our patients. But on none of these occasions, when we went through the records and spoke to the nurses and doctors concerned, had we missed anything. If somebody is determined to commit suicide, they will. They are very good at covering up what they're planning to do because even if people have been seriously depressed, once they've made up their mind that they're going to do it, their apparent mood lightens quite a lot.

I certainly became more aware of the huge variety of human behaviour and sometimes what its triggers were and sometimes there weren't any apparent triggers at all. Life in the Navy was relatively black and white. Life at The Priory was a multi-coloured spectrum. You never knew what each day was going to bring. I don't think quiet days existed at The Priory.

By 1995 we were talking to Westminster Healthcare about merging the companies and therefore the company could be deemed to be in a sale process, so there was nothing to stop outsiders making a bid for it. Indeed, we went public shortly afterwards.

Ian Reynolds [David Wakefield's deputy] continued to bid for the company and persuaded his backers, Mercury Development Capital (then Mercury Asset Management), to put the highest bid on the table. Other companies had been interested but pulled out as time went by and, at the suggestion of Richard Conte, I raised a Management Buy Out of my own, backed by HSBC. But Ian Reynolds managed to persuade Mercury (who seemed to be very keen to get The Priory Group) to pay a silly price and of course eventually they won. HSBC, quite rightly, were not prepared to pay the price. And as quickly became clear, Mercury overpaid, because they got rid of it a year later and hadn't really made any money out of it.

So the guy I had hired as my deputy was in effect plotting against me. I was very sad not to be the successful owner of the new business, which could then have continued as it had done before, and to be leaving the Group, which had been my life for 14 years.

But equally, I was glad that HSBC weren't prepared to pay a silly price because the pressure of running the Group to pay it back would have been absolutely intolerable. I'm usually pretty much an optimist and I think I was able to see that once the inevitable was there, I could do other things, which I've been very happy doing.

I had already been a Trustee of the HIV Hospice, the London Lighthouse, since 1994. I became the Vice Chairman of Lighthouse in '96, Chairman in '98, and in 2000 I merged it with the Terrence Higgins Trust. Then I became Chairman of the Terrence Higgins Trust until my period of office came to an end at the end of 2006.

I have been incredibly fortunate. My life has been divided into three quite distinct blocks: the Navy, The Priory, and now a series of non-exec directorships and chairmanships. They have all been hugely enjoyable, quite different and very satisfying. In some ways I can look back and say that's pretty much a model career; to have had the opportunity of that amount of variety and stimulation."

My son wanted to know more about me and his biological family (he had met his granny, aunt and uncle as a babe but of course didn't remember).

I told him that his grandfather (my Dad) had died when I was six and his aunt (my sister Susan) had been living in the States since I was eleven. When my brother Jim got married, that left just Mum and me at home. This wasn't an ideal arrangement because we didn't get on too well.

I was something of a mistake, arriving twelve years after Sue and ten years after Jim. When Mum realised she was pregnant again at the age of forty-three, she evidently asked Dad, "What will we do, Cecil?" and he replied, "We'll welcome the little stranger."

My brother was an Eton Chorister, I explained to Rob, and my sister attended a local convent. We were a very musical, two piano family. Susan played the piano and cello and Jim played the organ, piano, double bass, clarinet, flute and bassoon!

My fate was ballet school. Mum was one of the pianists at the school and I think her thwarted desire to dance as a child was to be realised through me because although Sue and Jim danced too, they weren't pushed to the same extent.

Dance classes began when I was two and by the age of four, I was attending ballet school full-time. Based in a large Victorian house in Buckinghamshire, the school occupied four floors overflowing with children, teachers, pianists and helpers.

Piano music wafted into every corner of my life. At school, wherever I was it accompanied me. And at home someone was usually playing and I would be allowed to stay up for occasional evening soirees, when such budding musicians as Benjamin Zander (to become Conductor of the Boston Philharmonic) would play his cello.

When I was six, and Mum told me I was to have piano lessons, I cried bitterly. I knew I would never be as good as my sister and brother. They seemed to share a world of musicality that I could never enter. They went to the piano with eager fingers and quick minds; I approached it with dread. I also knew how much practice they did and I just wanted to play with friends after school. But I needed Mum's approval and there would be a hiding if I didn't obey.

I was sent to the same piano teacher as Sue and Jim. He was a grey-haired giant with huge fingers. He used to touch me, patting in time with the music or stroking me during the slow bits. This made me play all the wrong notes. Later, as I began to develop breasts, he beat time on them and said "Ah yes, coming along nicely". Red-faced, I would race through the pieces to get them over and done with.

It seems incredible now that I didn't tell anyone; I probably felt it was somehow my fault. However, one day I put my foot down and told Mum I was never going back. I didn't tell her why and she was exceedingly angry. Mum is the only person I have ever fought with, physically. Unfortunately, another music teacher was soon found but at least she was a spinster and safe.

I was reasonable at the piano – I won some cups and was said to play with great feeling but I was awful at sight-reading – it took me ages to learn a piece. My Dad used to play by ear but had always regretted not being able to read music so Mum presented a cup to the local arts festival when he died. The Cecil S. White cup - a brand new class: sight-reading. She entered me for the class, perhaps hoping to shock me into improvement.

You had to wait out of earshot before your turn so that you didn't hear the efforts of the other contestants. Fear of the inevitable made me tremble as I approached the menacing piano. *The Whites are such a talented family*, I chided myself, *it says so in the papers, and now I'm going to shame us all*. And that is exactly what I did; in a hall full of people I surely besmirched my father's name.

Mum died three years before my son re-entered my life and so by the time I was relating this to him, I had come to terms with both sides of her; the fine pianist, who was an ambitious perfectionist, and the obsessive, who stayed up all night cleaning. For me, one of the most excruciating side effects of her obsessions was that if Mum wasn't required to play the piano for a few minutes in ballet class, her head would fall forward in slumber. Seeing this, I would dread the moment the music had to resume. The moment when the teacher would count her in - "And..." - and nothing would happen. "AND one and two..." and Mum would come to with a start, and I would flinch at the sniggers around me.

Nowadays, Mum would be recognised as suffering from obsessive-compulsive disorder (OCD). I would come down in the mornings and find her slumped in a chair in front of the electric fire, exhausted. It wasn't until I started staying with friends at weekends that I realised everyone's Mum didn't stay up all night cleaning. The fact that she never went to bed could beg the question, how was I ever conceived? I'm told that the neighbours called me 'the landing baby', the inference being that Dad had caught Mum at the top of the stairs and I was the result.

The aftermath of her self-destructive behaviour was that she had a stroke, leaving her paralysed down one side. It happened some months after Jim married, on the coldest, snowiest February night in memory. I had come home early from a dance rehearsal and found her on the kitchen floor. Had I returned at the usual time, we were told, she would have been dead. In hospital, the staff couldn't understand why she slept for days and days. I think she was catching up.

During Mum's time in hospital, her youngest brother visited from Newcastle. Of all her five brothers, Uncle Lindsay was the best. He had a lilting Scottish accent, never forgot my birthday, and seemed to have a soft spot for me. He was an important father figure.

I hadn't seen him since my brother's wedding some months earlier and after the hospital visit he came back to the house until it was time to catch his train. He asked to see my photograph album and sat companionably close. He kept breaking off from looking at the photos to look at me and said I was a beautiful sixteen year-old. I thought that was nice; praise from him made me glow.

But then things went wrong. He put his hand on my leg and leaned over to kiss me on the mouth. I was confused and made an excuse to leave the room but he was right behind me. He pinned me against the wall and tried to kiss me again. Ducking under his arms, I retreated to the kitchen. He came too and held me and forced his tongue into my mouth and one of his teeth must have been false because it clicked. My heart pounded in my head as I rushed back into the hall, and pulled against him as he tried to force me up the stairs.

At last I broke free and went for the front door, grabbing my coat. I was desperate not to cry and managed to announce that we had to leave for the station right away, even though it was an hour too early. I waited by the open door, my head down, shaking with fright. He seemed to get control of himself yet kept repeating that he adored me and would 'phone me every day and could he write to me? I shook my head and hurried blindly to the station with him making polite conversation at my side. On the walk back, I couldn't stop the tears. He phoned that evening. I was polite but said I didn't wish to speak to him.

When Mum came home, I didn't have the maturity or grit to deal with a depressed stroke victim. Maybe the worst thing was that I didn't seem to have the love. My relationship with Mum had always been an uneasy one; packed with push on her part and rebellion on mine. So our past did not equip us well for our present.

At the age of 59, her life as a capable and obsessional workaholic was over. My emotions were so chaotic that I couldn't accommodate hers. And hers must have been screaming at the indignity of being struck down. After work I'd go home to the results of her frustrated domestic efforts and begin the clearing up, cooking and washing. At night she had a bell to ring and I had to be awake when she visited the toilet. When she fell, I couldn't lift her so would fetch a neighbour. Bells always seemed to be ringing — if not in reality then in my dreams. After about nine weeks I was prescribed sleeping pills; I felt depressed and trapped.

The Department of Social Security advised me to leave home. I was astounded. Family disloyalty was surely what this amounted to, with Jim newly married and Susan in the States. But I found a room to rent nearby, collected some clothes, and made my escape. My survival instinct must have outweighed my guilt. My brother arranged for Mum to have live-in help. It was a bleak time for us all.

It was at this highly charged juncture that I met Bob. He was a photographer where I worked and he offered me lifts when he saw me walking. He was full of cheerful chat and friendly interest, and these brief interludes, with drinks at country pubs, plucked me out of sadness. They also filled me with yearning for attention and affection.

What happened next is nothing if not predictable: pregnancy. It is no excuse but I was a virgin and clueless, whereas Bob was 10 years older, should have known better, and turned out to be married.

He left his wife of one year; we lived in rented rooms and then went to live with Mum. This meant that we could save for our own place and that I could look after her again. She was still terribly depressed and one morning I came down to find her sawing at her wrist with the bread knife. She was doing it over the sink; she wouldn't want to make a mess.

So it was into this broken, complex family that I had welcomed Rob. It must have been alarming to hear all that stuff, and in a letter the following day, I apologised:

> "…Thank you so much for this weekend. Being with you seems like such a miracle and makes me so happy. Sometimes I worry that I'll wake up and it will all have been a dream. Now, too, I'm worrying that I told you too much yesterday and am cross with myself and hope you're not too appalled…"

What I also had to get across to Rob was that despite all my negative feelings about being forced into music, despite the hidings and my stupidity about reading the notes at speed, I now knew how privileged I had been. My early and sustained exposure to music had been the greatest possible gift.

9
Gatekeepers of the Mind

Free of the restraints of the NHS, Priory Consultants relished the liberty of actually spending time with patients. They were all at the top of their game and fulfilling their own areas of clinical responsibility. Any pressure from the administration merely augmented their bond as a team. They just got on with it.

Some people say that psychiatrists can be on the strange side. I confess I did wonder if, in the interests of helping a patient, they didn't occasionally tiptoe over that thin line between sanity and madness. But for the most part, Priory shrinks seemed remarkably normal to me.

It must surely be the relationship that forms between psychiatrist and patient - a beneficial blend of psychotherapy and medication - that makes the relationship so successful. DK's view was that psychiatry is an art, not a science, and he selected consultants who were healers, with natural empathy, genuineness and warmth. One thing is for sure: none of them were average.

Dr John Cobb, Consultant Psychiatrist
Priory Years: 1985 – 2004

"Desmond Kelly knew me pretty well because we overlapped at St George's and when he left there for The Priory, we kept in touch. I remember rather vividly a meeting at the Maudsley Hospital, when I was presenting a paper about behaviour therapy in agoraphobia where there are marital problems - funny how you remember the detail! Desmond was in the audience and asked me afterwards if I'd like to work at The Priory.

I was discontented with George's at the time so it all slotted together, as these things sometimes do in life. I had concerns about moving, partly because of security, having three kids and a mortgage, and it felt like a big step for me. But David Wakefield [Hospital Director] was enormously helpful and influential.

Years before, I'd actually done a locum with Dr William Sargant at The Priory. I was doing research at the Maudsley and twice a week got the bus to do ward rounds for Will Sargant on the Narcosis Unit. The patients were put to sleep for 3 weeks, given ECT, and a complicated combination of drugs. I was amazed by what I saw on that unit. Of course Sargant was extraordinary and very charismatic. He almost bullied the patients into getting better: 'You *will* get better! You have had the best treatment in the world!'

John Flood was the Medical Director then, a jolly Irishman, very genial and red faced, but the place was a bit chaotic in those days. Wine was always served at the Monday lunches and most of the Consultants would play golf in the afternoon. I thought *gosh, this is the other side of psychiatry!* It was like a gentleman's club.

Desmond introduced the academic element, which made it really appealing to me because it was bringing together two streams.

St George's was very academic but Springfield Hospital, where I was based, was an awful old asylum. It was one of the things I noticed at The Priory – there wasn't a smell of disinfectant and cooked cabbage. I forgot what it had been like at Springfield and when I went back there to give a lecture six months later, it hit me - *how could I have worked here for 7 years?*

So The Priory was a clean, wholesome, pleasant place to be. Eric Shur came to visit before he started working there and said, 'John, the thing I notice when I come here is that you always seem so happy and so proud of the place.' That's how it was.

It was peaceful too. The thing about NHS wards was the noise; the clanking, banging, shouting, almost unnecessary noise, and the fact that there were no carpets on the floor. People would say 'If you're not mad when you get admitted here, when you've been here for a week you'll certainly be mad.'

At The Priory I remember one of my patients saying, 'The thing about The Priory, which is different to any treatment I've had before, is that you're not a 'case' with a diagnosis, you're a human being.' And of course there were wonderful nurses like Renée and Camille, and the Matron Betty Naudeer, who saw every patient every day.

When Desmond was talking about getting somebody new on the staff he'd say, 'I'd like to welcome on board...'. I think he saw himself as the captain of the ship. And in a way that's what that place needs; somebody at the top, with other people getting on with their roles. So there wasn't any backstabbing or people trying to compete with one another. Initially, we were paid a generous retainer, but that meant we weren't paid for looking after inpatients. Whether you had one inpatient or eight, you were paid the same. So what happened was that people tended to be quite happy about sharing out inpatients and everybody in the end looked after about the same number. Each of the Consultants was on call one night a week and one weekend in four. One looks back on those times and think they were the good old days.

The Thursday clinical meetings were well attended and were seen as the academic central point of the week. Again there was an atmosphere which was different to the NHS. The patients were included as an integral part of the meeting and had their say along with everyone else.

Sometimes the unexpected would occur. One time the Eating Disorder Unit presented a girl as a great success. She had been at death's door this young lass; down to 3½ stone but she had been in treatment for 4 or 5 months and was very well. She looked good, was back to 8 stone, was well balanced and getting on with her family, who were there with her. We used to ask the patient questions, and somebody said 'Tell us about your plans. What are you going to do when you leave the hospital?' She looked him straight in the eye and said 'I'm going to lose weight.' There were gasps all round.

Another one was a lovely old lady from a well-heeled family, who had been in the alcohol unit and done extremely well. She was full of good intentions, had definitely given up drink and had seen the damage it had done. Her husband was there and somebody asked him 'How do you think your wife has done? Has she really given up?' He said, 'Well, I suppose so, up to a point. Of course she still has wine with dinner.' She turned on him and said 'Having wine with dinner is *not* drinking.'

There was a very nice schizophrenic lady who was admitted under section [Section of the Mental Health Act] and made a run for it. She went through reception and I happened to be there and could see the nurses were following but she was a fast and fit young lady. I went after her and rugby tackled her on the lawn. There was great applause from the people around! Subsequently she said, 'You probably saved my life because I was heading for the railway line'. That's what she was after: to jump off Barnes Bridge. I must add that she remains my patient to this day and sends me Christmas cards without fail. So much for empathy, genuineness and warmth for establishing rapport!

I was the Clinical Tutor from 1986 to 1992 and had a lot of informal clinical interaction with Registrars too. We would have lunch together during the week (not just on Mondays) and would have tea on the wards quite often with the nurses. Not a ward round or a meeting but an informal chat. That was very constructive and the Pharmacist, Virginia Jervis, used to take a good part in that.

I enjoyed teaching and the Registrars were of a high calibre, keen and receptive. I ran quite a number of seminars for them and they took an active part. They said that there wasn't a stereotypical Priory Consultant; that we all had our strengths and weaknesses and things to say, some of which were brilliant and some of which seemed to be nonsense.

Having said that, one of the reasons I came to The Priory was because I had been teaching about three days a week at St George's. I was a Senior Lecturer and what they called a Peripatetic Tutor, going round from one hospital to another, teaching juniors. I had really had a belly full of teaching. So I didn't particularly want to come to The Priory and repeat what I had been doing at George's. I actually wanted to do some patient work.

My interest in obsessive-compulsive disorder (OCD) began when I was sitting having a cup of coffee in the canteen at the Maudsley one day. I had just got my

MRCPsych and Professor Isaac Marks came up and said how about doing some research on OCD? I liked Isaac and was very pleased to have the offer. I spent two years with a Medical Research Council grant on the use of either clomipramine or behaviour therapy as a treatment for OCD.

I was aware that psychosurgery for OCD was going on and had an open mind about it. When I came to The Priory, I saw some very impressive results with Desmond's patients so I started putting my patients through the same procedure. The curious thing is – although I haven't got the statistics to prove this – I don't think my patients did anything like as well as Desmond's patients, despite their follow up being exactly the same. Maybe I got referred more difficult patients than he did!

Behaviour therapy works. It's explicit, understandable and people know what they're getting into. I like it because it's collaborative. You feel you're working with the patient rather than doing something to them. I still see quite a number of obsessional patients. Professor Sir Aubrey Lewis, head of the Maudsley Hospital where I trained, was a great writer about OCD and all psychiatry, and he said 'He who can understand the mystery of obsessive-compulsive disorder will understand human nature itself.' And we all have it you know, little checking rituals; it is there in all of us.

The Thames Television series *A Problem Aired* was one of the good things that came out of being Clinical Tutor. A lady rang The Priory and said she wanted to do a television series about psychological treatment, counselling, and could she come and have a chat? I had lunch with her in the dining room and was quite sceptical. I said I didn't think any consultant would want to do it and thought I'd put her off. A week later she phoned again to say she was going to send me the details of a programme, they would advertise to get the patients, and would I do it? I said 'Oh! I'm not sure!' But there's always been a little hidden showman in me.

It was entirely unscripted, it was live, and I had not met the patients. Researchers met them and wrote reports and I had the final veto. When I shook hands (and people used to joke about the way I seemed to be leaning out as if to grope them), it was because I'd never met them before.

I insisted that I didn't want the interview to be interrupted with advertisements and the maximum they could run anything in those days without an ad was 23½ minutes. I had a bug in the ear telling me 'five minutes', 'three minutes to go', and then they'd be counting down.

During one of the first programmes I thought I was doing really well, took a sip of water and then realised I couldn't swallow it! I used to try and control my nerves and realised after that experience that if I do that, it actually goes into my throat. So I can appear to be very calm but my throat is seizing up.

Some of the programmes went very well; some went badly. So it wasn't just showing someone doing something brilliantly, it was someone at work. There was one lady who was a real dragon and I got nowhere. In fact I was wishing they'd turn the cameras off. The cameramen used to give me feedback afterwards and on this occasion it was: 'Phew Doc, she 'ad you for breakfast!'

It got to the point where I was recognised quite a bit. A cab driver said he was so pleased to see me because he'd never had anybody famous in his cab before. And when I stopped at lights, a guy in the car beside me drew a television in the air and pointed at me, and at Munich Airport someone in the passport queue said 'I know you!' It was fun. The programme ran for about four years but one of the last things Margaret Thatcher did was to take the franchise away from Thames Television.

I often set patients books to read. I say I'd like you to read this poem or go and see that opera or film. It's all there really; you don't need psychiatric textbooks. You need the psychiatric knowledge first of all – the nuts and bolts – but having got a good orthodox training you can soften that and make it more human by introducing literature and art.

I use quite a lot of imagery - 'I want you to go and see a Caravaggio at the National Gallery and see whether it says anything to you.' Great stuff; it makes it very interesting for the patient and for me.

If you're asking is there a kind of patient I dread, the answer is, not now. There certainly was when I started but I think it's all to do with your own psyche and if you're finding a patient in some way unattractive or difficult, it's usually something in yourself and not something in the patient. And I've always had good people to supervise me or discuss things with. I still see someone. No, what I've found difficult is some colleagues and administrators!

So I would say that initially, certainly for the first ten years or so, The Priory was the most enjoyable part of my psychiatric career. And in a way we've got Desmond to thank for that – because he was a strong, organised, naval officer-type leader, who ran a good ship.

Now, I enjoy working three days a week, it keeps me active and patients getting better is always a source of delight."

Another anecdote from John:

No case to answer
"A schizophrenic patient had stopped his medication and was getting more and more crazy, and got the idea - I must see Dr Cobb. He got in his car, drove through Richmond Park at 80 miles an hour, screamed into The Priory drive and slammed the brakes on.

The police had been alerted to something strange so two police cars followed him in. He ran into The Priory and because he'd been an inpatient he knew the place. He was running round the corridors one way and the police the other, like something from a French farce.

Eventually he ended up in my office, followed by exhausted policemen. 'Are you all right, sir?' they asked. 'Yes fine, we're just talking about it,' I said. Amazingly, they didn't charge him!"

Dr Jeanie Speirs, Consultant Psychiatrist
Priory Years: 1989 – ongoing

> Jeanie Speirs talked about her experience of The Priory immediately after the retirement tea party for Dr Eric Shur, a treasured consultant colleague she had worked with closely. Her mind was full of him and, as ever, she was extremely modest about her own achievements.

"This is a momentous day. We'll miss Eric a lot. He's funny, erudite and very reliable. Uniquely, he and I have done 'ward rounds' together every Monday at 9.15am for more than 20 years – nothing has ever got in the way of them. If he's away or I'm away we cover each other. It has been a way of having clinical audit and informed cover. I've been able to say this patient has now been on so much of something for three weeks, do you think I should increase it or should I wait or add anything else? And it's really nice to have that kind of sounding board. We sit in here with the junior doctor and nurse for the ward that we're talking about, together with our link therapists. So we get feedback from the therapists, feedback from the ward, and then we present the patients to each other. We will miss Eric a lot.

I came here in October 1989. I didn't really think about being the only female Consultant when I started because I knew Saeed Islam and Eric Shur very well from Westminster Hospital days (we were all junior doctors there) so it just seemed like being with two old friends and then making new ones and everyone was incredibly friendly. Desmond Kelly was very welcoming too. He held the whole place together; he was very cohesive.

I had done quite a lot of psychotherapy and also an analytical training in the Eighties. I had the occasional psychoanalytical patient, with supervision, but never did that all day every day. And coming to The Priory, because there are so many good therapists here, one was just the consultant in charge. I mostly use a cognitive type of therapy but sometimes use a more psychodynamic approach. There were a few patients who wanted to see a female psychiatrist, when colleagues (as mere males) weren't good enough! So that helped me build my practice.

I specialise now in perinatal work [the period just before or just after birth] but when I started here I was more into psychotherapy and sexual therapy. I didn't particularly like the latter, I must say, I found it rather a seedy subject quite frankly! But, for example, the treatment for impotence has changed and is taken care of more by urologists than psychiatrists. And of course Viagra is now available. Before, one used psychological methods, such as Masters and Johnson. I think those behavioural methods do work but people quite often get their confidence back via Viagra and then they're all right anyway.

I got into perinatal work partly because my sister-in-law had post-natal problems but I didn't recognise it because I hadn't done any psychiatry by then. I subsequently went to a conference and there was quite a bit on it and I thought it very interesting and started to pursue it.

Postnatal treatment is almost easier than perinatal treatment, because it's an acute situation you're dealing with. The most difficult thing is when somebody comes along and says 'I've got bipolar [a severe condition in which patients swing from deep depression into euphoria], I'm on lithium carbonate and sodium valproate, and I'm thinking about becoming pregnant. What should I do?' I have a patient at the moment who when she said she wanted a baby, the only thing I could think about was retiring! Hopefully I looked as though I was going to try and facilitate it. So I've set it all up and there's a Plan A and Plan B. For Plan A she wants to try and be medication-free in the first trimester. If that doesn't work, we go to Plan B.

When women are on loads of medication and are 40 and say they want to have a baby, you simply haven't got time to test out different scenarios. And by that stage the risks of an abnormal pregnancy are far higher, based on age alone. So you have a different number of statistics to weigh up. But fingers crossed I've seen quite a few people through on rather noxious substances, talking about it throughout, and liaising with the obstetricians. It's a very good feeling when somebody who has been tortured by their symptoms responds to medication and is feeling much better.

I enjoy anything to do with colleagues. One of the highlights of the week is the Thursday Case Conference – I've always liked that and it's a great tradition. Sometimes one can't get to it but when Desmond was around it was a three line whip! One was there, end of story! And actually that was a very good thing. I think it was even written into my original contract. It's really important for Continuous Professional Development (CPD) too because you have to have external and internal points. An hour's case conference a week fulfils most of the internal points you need, in a wonderfully convenient way.

When Desmond asked me to be the Medical Student Tutor I was a bit daunted but I wouldn't have said no. I felt a certain honour in being asked and definitely wouldn't have been pulling my weight as part of the peer group if I hadn't taken it on. We all took on various roles and it was important to get given a role and to do one's very best at it. Actually, it was most enjoyable.

It was a new venture so I had to look at what was required and go to meetings at University College London (UCL) to find out what students were expected to experience during their four week placements. We were able to provide practically all they required, in terms of teaching, case conferences, clerking and presenting patients. The only things we weren't able to offer were outpatient and community work. But they received excellent experience of acute psychiatry.

Then it was about everyone getting used to the concept that there were medical students around. All students had to sign a confidentiality form. Clearly there has to be confidentiality with all patients, whoever they are, but the temptation to talk to others is greater if the patient is well-known. It was one of the biggest things I emphasised, the Hippocratic oath - the reasons for being struck off the Medical Register.

I'm quite obsessional actually, I'm sure it drives my husband mad! I might have been good at organising timetables and if colleagues didn't turn up for their teaching slots, I would follow that up. If they were consistently unreliable, I took them off the timetable, because that's hopeless. I did teaching slots as well as their inductions, evaluations and feedback.

Quite a few consultant colleagues took on teaching slots. On their feedback forms students had to say if there was a particular teacher who was good and if somebody got mentioned more than anybody else, they got a special accolade.

Eric Shur was one of them. If a student hadn't produced a case to present, which is what they're meant to do, Eric acted out the patient. He climbed under the desk and the dismayed students had to coax him out, while he would be looking up, worrying about cameras and being persecuted! They would remember the Consultant who crawled around under the desk, I'm sure, and remember what came after that, how to elicit whether he was hearing voices and so on. Wonderful teaching!

Latterly, the exams at University College Hospital have been Objective Structured Clinical Examinations (OSCEs) and very scary for the students. There are 30 stations in a big room and a bell goes every three minutes and they go from one station to the next. At each station there is something they have to answer, and examiners like me who supervise the situation and do the marking. The marking instructions are really clear so its very fair and that's the whole point: the student has either said something or they haven't.

For instance, a station could have an audio video set and the student comes in, puts the headphones on and looks at an interview of a psychiatrist and a patient. On their sheet of paper they have to fill in the mental state, the appearance, the mood, perceptions, delusions, insight, cognitive state etc. While the next student is watching, you're marking the last student. There are also actors pretending to be patients.

I believe the students thought The Priory was a wonderful placement. We got fantastic feedback and always came up trumps because they got a lot of consultant input and they were valued.

Here we are in the private sector, having managed to get teaching hospital status: that is extremely unusual. Everyone realises how unique it is, how valuable, and what a privilege it is. So we welcome students rather than thinking *oh no, there are students coming onto the ward, what a nuisance.* The students symbolise an achievement.

Away from work, I have a great passion for shells. We've just been to East Africa and collected lots of shells. I'm not too bothered about what kind of shell it is; it's the shape and colour that matters for me. You're not really meant to take them off the beach but I do pick tiny ones occasionally without being too indiscreet.

I look forward to having an evening at home with nice things to eat and drink. We've found a really nice place to be in the country. I don't know how we managed to find that place. It sort of happened without too much real research and it's only since we've been there that we've realised just how right it is. So I stay in town two nights a week. And for my husband, he is now only 7 miles from an airfield where he keeps his little plane. Sometimes I'll phone him and he'll say 'I'm on the Isle of Wight having a cup of tea.'"

Dr Eric Shur, Consultant Psychiatrist & Deputy Medical Director
Priory Years: 1990 – 2010

> A few days after his retirement, Dr Shur and I arranged to meet at Dr Kelly's home, around the corner from The Priory. I noticed that Eric kept using the phrase "when I came over…" and that was how it felt to him, his move from the NHS to the private sector.

"The first job I ever had in this country, when I arrived from South Africa in 1976, was as Senior House Officer for Dr Peter Dally [an international expert in eating disorders]. He had a unit at All Saints' Hospital in Lambeth. So I worked with his eating disorder patients and found them fascinating. I also found Peter to be a very charismatic figure. It has been shown that the thing that determines which speciality students go into is when they come across a really charismatic teacher. So he kind of hooked me in. He and Professor Arthur Crisp are the people who put eating disorders on the map in this country.

I then worked for Professor Gerald Russell, who also made a major contribution to eating disorders and ran a programme at the Maudsley Hospital. I worked on his unit for six months as a Senior House Officer, and then became his Lecturer for two years. So I worked on his unit for two years doing research and some clinical work and I got to be quite good at it I think.

The difficulty with eating disorders is that people die. It has the highest mortality rate of all the psychiatric disorders. So you get these young (usually girls), who will die occasionally, and that was very very difficult.

But other than that I found it a most fascinating field because there's something in it for everybody. It has a biological basis, almost certainly; the family dynamics are very important; there are major cultural elements and lots of psychological aspects. It's got psychotherapy, medical treatments, family therapy, social intervention, and that's why you have to have a team and I like the multi-disciplinary team approach.

My decision to go from the NHS into private practice was prompted by a call from Dr Saeed Islam actually. He said "We have a vacancy at The Priory do you want to come?" I said "Oh no, I've just been appointed as a Consultant three years ago, I've got too much to do". He said "Just come and have a look at the place." I made my mind up in 2 days! I'm quite an impulsive person in that way. When I came over from South Africa to England, I came on holiday, a trip around Europe, and decided to stay, just like that. So all the big decisions in my life have been rather impulsive I suppose.

It was a bit of a leap into the unknown. In those days it was quite unfashionable to be in private practice. It was seen as something really bad. Private medicine was a very small part of medicine, and still is really, but it was socially unacceptable in the NHS. So it was quite a big step to take.

Some disapproved; the people who had left-wing leanings certainly did. The professor I worked for, who believed in socialised medicine, was very anti at the beginning. Actually he is now a Visiting Consultant at The Priory. When I left the NHS, some of the team were really angry with me, nurses and psychologists and so on. Partly because they felt I was leaving them in the lurch, and partly because they disapproved of what I was doing. But I think a lot of them were envious as well.

Desmond called me a few weeks before I started: 'We need a Deputy Medical Director. Would you be willing to take it on?' I said 'OK.' Then he phoned a week later and said 'Would you be willing to be the Clinical Tutor?' I should have said 'Hang on, let me get my feet under the desk and think about it.' But I said, 'OK.'

So apart from a time when others took over for a couple of years, I was the Clinical Tutor throughout my time at The Priory. I loved working with the junior doctors, which I had done before in the NHS, when I was the Tutor to Senior Registrars. There was also quite a lot of work from time to time - I remember one year we had 250 applicants for one post. So 250 CVs arrived on my desk and I had to shortlist in 4-5 days.

I enjoy being second in command so I liked the Deputy role. It wasn't very arduous – just covering for the Medical Director when he was away and talking things over as appropriate.

One difference in the private sector was the relative lack of bureaucracy and red tape. Unfortunately, in latter years its getting more and more NHS-like as the number of hospitals has grown, edicts from head office, clinical governance. But when I came to The Priory you had nearly complete freedom of clinical practice, which was wonderful. You weren't constrained by managers telling you what you could and couldn't do.

The other main difference of course was that in the private sector you spend 90% of your time treating patients. Whereas when I was in the NHS I probably spent 20% of my time with patients. And there were usually layers of junior doctors between me and the patients. At one time I had an SHO, a Registrar, and a Senior Registrar, so that filters out most of the problems. I felt that I was only really clinically challenged when I went into private practice.

There was a really good morale at The Priory. Everybody seemed happy, they knew what they were doing, there was a tremendous feeling of camaraderie, team spirit. In those days we had a system where you weren't paid a fee for service so we got paid an excellent salary. Whether you had one or two or ten patients, you got paid the same. That meant that we were all kind of equal, it was more like a socialist network in the hospital. And if one of us was a bit overloaded, we'd help each other.

When I joined there were three hospitals, of which Roehampton was the biggest, owned by an American family, the Contes. Yes they wanted to make a profit (and they did) but they were actually somewhat altruistic, I felt. They were Anglophiles, and very proud of the place and of what we were doing. It was like a little family, everybody knew everybody else and it was a very nice atmosphere.

Once a week I used to teach the junior doctors presentation skills. I used to try and help them to learn how to present a case properly. They came one day and they hadn't got a case. So I said 'I tell you what, I will be the patient, and I want you to do a mental state on me and then we'll discuss it afterwards.'

I thought, *I'll do a paranoid psychosis*, and I really got into it. I started by seeming incredibly nervous, then he asked me a question in a sharp way and I jumped off my chair, crawled under my desk and wouldn't come out. I wanted him to try and relax me and try and talk me down so that I would come out. And he did to some extent, and I came out. Then I said 'OK, now let's do a mental state examination. Present me with the case'. For some reason they really liked this and that year voted me the best psychiatric teacher in the medical school.

I used to comment on their appearance, the way they sat, their eye contact, and hand movements. That went down well because nobody had talked to them about that sort of thing before.

I remember when I was at the Maudsley, I had to organise mock exams for the Registrars. They would come in and examine the patient and present the case to two examiners, and these were real examiners for membership of the Royal College of Psychiatrists. And I videotaped the whole thing. I then took the video tapes and gave them to examiners and got them to watch it for two minutes and asked them to rate the candidate after two minutes.

Then I got them to watch the whole tape, about 20 minutes, and then rate them again. And to my amazement, hardly any of them changed their minds. That meant they had made their minds up in the first two minutes about whether this person was going to pass or fail. Then what they would do, once they had made their minds up, was just gather information to confirm that hypothesis. So it occurred to me that it must be something about the way they were sitting, the way they were speaking, their eye contact, their body language, which is actually more important than what they're saying. So I put this to them and said they had to come across as competent, confident, and impress the examiner in those first two minutes.

Obviously it's good to have a sense of humour, it keeps you going. But I think most psychiatrists have a dark side to them, otherwise they wouldn't do it. So it's a question of keeping that dark side under control and keeping a good sense of humour the rest of the time. I wouldn't say it's essential. It just makes you more pleasant to be around, especially as a colleague. And your patients like it too, definitely. I did have some good laughs with my patients.

I learnt an enormous amount from the clinical case conferences. I was really impressed with the clinical acumen of the people at The Priory, which was far superior to most other consultants I'd seen outside The Priory, in terms of their clinical abilities. Before I came over, most of the people I knew, professors and so on, were good academics but they weren't that good as clinicians on the whole.

The consultants at The Priory were not quoting academic papers at you left, right and centre, but they were able to get to the nub of the clinical cause and understand the patient and empathise and make some very good interventions.

And we used to have splendid seminars, with important speakers. I remember getting 150 people and we had an overflow room with a television link. The Priory was one of the first to do these seminars. People even recently have said to me, 'I remember those seminars, they were fantastic, why don't you do more of those?'

I have always found my patients much more interesting than anything else. You could go to a psychological thriller but it would be nothing compared to the stories your patients were telling you. And they were generally really nice people. So I loved that side of it. I also liked the feeling of everybody working together. I loved The Priory – the building, the grounds. My office was spectacular, with a lovely view.

I started going to the gym at The Priory about 15 years ago and kept it up virtually twice a week for about 15 years without fail. They very kindly let me use the gym after hours. That was really important to me and I was pleased that I could do that, it made a big difference. I had it to myself - me and my trainer - we used to go there at 7pm when I'd finished with patients.

So I've always had it in my mind to retire at least by 60, if not earlier. I may be wrong but I felt that there may be another side to me that's bursting to come out. I've felt that frequently during my life as a doctor, that there's another side of me. And I thought that if I retired maybe that would come out. We will see! I'm going to study the History of Art.

I am just very thankful that I got to The Priory, and that Saeed phoned me up that day. I have learned a huge amount and I couldn't have worked at a better place or with nicer people. So no regrets."

See more from Eric in the *Time Out* chapter.

Dr Mark Collins, Consultant Psychiatrist
Priory Years: 1991 – ongoing

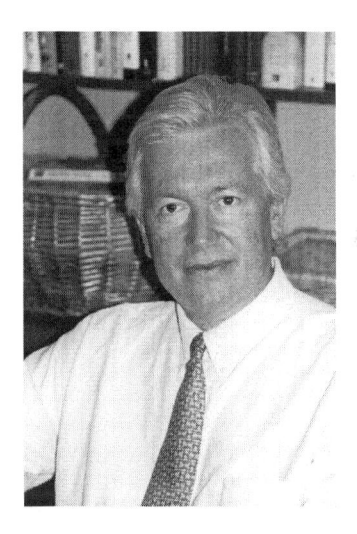

"I grew up in a lovely house just by St Paul's Cathedral, built by Sir Christopher Wren. It was actually a tied cottage, in the sense that it went with the job of Canon of St Paul's, which is what my father was. I discovered as an adult that the house was the exact location of the Royal College of Physicians before the Great Fire of London. So where I played in my nursery was where the physician William Harvey had played with his veins and then written his celebrated treatise describing the circulation of blood. The house was very close to St Bartholomew's Hospital and we had a medical student lodger (the daughter of friends of my parents) and she had a skeleton in her bedroom. At the age of 4, I was completely fascinated by this and announced, 'I'm going to be a doctor.'

I had every intention of being a physician and was lucky enough to get honours in the final exams, the only one in my year who did (I'm showing off!) and was very much set on a career in medicine. I passed the MRCP [Membership of the Royal College of Physicians], went to America for three years and did neurology training there.

But I found myself increasingly frustrated by the mechanics of physical medicine. I remember treating somebody with a heart attack and his poor wife came to me full of gratitude. I thought all I've really done is press button A then other things have followed. I was much more interested in what was going on for the patient psychologically and was increasingly drawn to the possibility of switching to psychiatry. I had a very close friend who himself was a psychiatrist and he was egging me on. And I had heard Professor Arthur Crisp lecture and he had been very charismatic.

So in the end I made this quantum leap. I gathered that if you wanted to do abstract research you went to the Maudsley; if you wanted to do hands-on psychiatry with a psychotherapy emphasis, you went to St George's. I was lucky enough to get on to the George's training rotation at a time when it was really excellent. I was Dr Peter Storey's last registrar before his retirement, an absolutely wonderful man.

When I was appointed to my consultant post at the NHS in January 1990, I didn't have a clue what private practice was about. Mind you, I had been part of Dr John Cobb's tutorial group when I was a trainee at St George's. His was the most hotly sought-after training group, and it was a great loss for George's when he went to The Priory. Peter Storey was a Visiting Consultant at The Priory too.

What happened was that once I became a consultant in Wandsworth, somebody from the Charter Clinic in Chelsea came to schmooze me: would I have a look around Charter? By complete coincidence, the day I visited was the day their medical director and associate medical director resigned. So they were suddenly without their two key medical people and asked if I would look after private patients who weren't assigned to a particular consultant. I learned on the hoof, met some GPs in the Chelsea area and gradually built up a practice.

After a year or two, Elizabeth Logie, the Hospital Relations Manager at The Priory, and Rob Swindlehurst, then the Hospital Director, took me out for a stunning dinner. Elizabeth made a strong pitch that it would be in my interests to be linked with The Priory because it was a good hospital and it was close geographically to my St George's connections. They offered me a part-time staff contract, which I accepted. That was 1991.

My private practice mushroomed and I was trying to be a diligent NHS doctor, which meant that I was doing all my NHS hours and trying to do private practice in the evenings and be a husband and father to three small children. Elizabeth again (I think in discussion behind the scenes with Desmond Kelly) offered me a full time post. I met Dr Kelly and was hugely impressed with him.

I thought he was a wonderful warm character. He was very concerned with appropriate standards of excellence and turning The Priory into a true teaching hospital with medical students and trainees.

After much agonising and soul searching – because I was actually very committed to the NHS – I made the decision that something had to give and it would be the NHS that was going. So I started full time at The Priory in September 1993.

In some respects it was, to me, quite extraordinarily like taking a step back in time. I remember telling my consultant colleagues – by the way I'll be having my multi-disciplinary ward round at such and such a time – and wondering why there was silence. One of them said 'Mark, I don't think you understand. In the NHS we have multi-disciplinary ward rounds with social workers and everyone. In private psychiatry the consultant decides what to do and then tells everyone else.'

Although that is a slight exaggeration, it was still more medico-centric than the NHS, not necessarily to anyone's disadvantage but it was certainly quite striking to walk into that culture. Some aspects struck me negatively and I was able to work towards their change, which is just natural evolution.

We were doing audit at The Priory before anybody else. It was standard practice and very healthy that we would take a round of case notes from one of our colleagues and discuss them in the group format. The Thursday clinical meetings were of huge educational value. Desmond Kelly ran them in a formal and structured way and each consultant after the presentation had to give an opinion.

I think, again, if I was the new boy tilting a bit, it was to introduce the idea that we might have more of a discussion rather than you simply declaring in your oracular way what your view is then moving on to the next person; that there should be a little to and fro and dialogue. A change that I may have contributed to over the early years was the idea that we would bring in other disciplines too, so that you would get the therapy department to present a patient, or the therapists from Galsworthy Lodge [addiction unit] to present.

I think the whole consultant body found it a bit difficult when I first arrived – whether that was to do with my personality or simply that they felt a little bit 'oh dear, he's talking about these things that go on in the NHS or in the addiction world' – it all seemed like a bit too much change too quickly perhaps. I'm the youngest child in my family so I'm used to poking slight fun at my elders, because that was my role at home. I think when I'm the new boy in school I don't meekly wait my turn to be called; I tend to make a bit of noise straight away. I think that dynamic was played out here.

I didn't know any of the consultants apart from Dr Cobb, but all of them were massively supportive. As an example, a year or two after I joined, I went on a skiing holiday for a week, and when I left the hospital I had 17 patients under my care. I ended up being off work for two months because I injured my back.

Everybody instantly stepped in. They divided my patients between them, did the work and allowed the consultant fees to be retained by me because they were aware of how difficult it might be without that. It was extremely gentlemanly and kind and I never forgot it.

My practice included quite a lot of patients with addiction problems. Galsworthy Lodge at that stage was overseen by David Craggs, he was the wise old man keeping a very light hand on the tiller. As he headed towards retirement, I became progressively more involved, and when he retired I took over.

Galsworthy Lodge was unlike anything in the NHS and streets ahead of most addiction therapy. However, nothing stays still and actually over time it became a bit the other way, a bit stuck in its past. It had not caught up with the developments in America. One of the things I got very involved in was introducing certain things into the Galsworthy programme that were becoming normal in the addiction field. For example today people with depression or Seasonal Affective Disorder (SAD) or trauma are simultaneously identified and treated, rather than just dealing with the addiction.

There was probably a bias towards alcohol treatment when I arrived. People still looked upon drug addicts as rather strange creatures, and that changed in the sense that we got much more in the way of addiction to other chemicals. Also, there was the beginning of the idea that you could have other addictions than chemical ones. You could have behavioural addictions too, so food, gambling and so on we started introducing. When I say 'we', I was certainly a little part of it. But I did get more involved with the counsellors and with the direction of the therapy programme.

My own view then, and now, is that to be a good psychiatrist it helps if you have a good medical background as well – more than just the standard house jobs. Neurology, particularly, gives you a real grounding. A sense of humour is an essential thing for the make up of a decent psychiatrist. You have to keep yourself sane because you have to be simultaneously very empathic to people who have a lot of pain, sadness, hurt, disturbed boundaries, while retaining your own sanity. One way of achieving that is to maintain a sense of humour.

Patients want lots of things but an important thing they want is to know that they're dealing with a human being. If you have a sense of humour, even in poignantly difficult times, and as long as it is applied appropriately, that's good. Inevitably in private psychiatric practice there's an intense depth of knowledge of that person and the relationship becomes quite important in the patient's life sometimes.

I really respect Desmond for all the huge work he did. It was an uphill struggle for a private institution to get in at an academic level. When I was a trainee at St George's, it was pretty left wing and they said over our dead bodies will we have trainees in private medicine. But Desmond persevered and got Charing Cross and University College Hospital rotations, a definite plus factor. Great research has come out of The Priory with trainees doing quite important papers. And that continues.

As time has evolved, I've developed an interest in trauma – both big T and little t trauma. Big T is post-traumatic stress disorder, one single terrible event, a car crash or a tsunami. Little t trauma is those events that may not be huge in someone else's life but in yours they are, and they're unresolved and they inform your behaviour. That's when I got interested in a particular treatment technique called EMDR – Eye Movement Desensitization Reprocessing[*].

Personally, I'm not keen to get too much into the celebrity side of things. Ruby Wax became a personal friend because my wife was doing a fundraiser for the charity Depression Alliance and Ruby (who I had been treating at the time) very sweetly agreed to come and talk. It was the late Nineties and she was prepared to be vociferous about her experiences of depression and her recovery from it, with her little twist of humour.

So my wife became friends with Ruby in that context and gradually that evolved into a collective friendship, and her children are not dissimilar ages to my children. I still try to maintain the boundary of occasionally advising Ruby on just the medication aspects of things but nothing more than that. And I prefer to keep my own profile below the parapet.

Ultimately, celebrities are normal people with the same issues as anybody else. They just happen to do a particular job that gets them into the media and I would say that is to a large extent a bit of a nightmare, being exposed to tabloid media. OK you can be cynical about career advancement moves but in general that invasion of privacy or the catapulting from so-called normality to suddenly having people fawning all over you and clicking cameras, is pretty horrid. I certainly don't envy people their celebrity.

In the Nineties, the delights were simply getting patients better, working together as teams, and pride in the hospital. Everybody had an investment in the institution, at all levels. People had their moans but there was a real sense of loyalty and respect for The Priory. Certainly in those days there hadn't been any of the tabloid negative publicity that seems to be an inevitable part of 21st century life in this country.

Desmond Kelly is a great fan of Transcendental Meditation and I try to do a little bit of that, easily once a day. Not TM as such but what you would broadly call meditation. I relax with my family – that's number one, always has been always

---

[*] EMDR is a powerful psychological method developed by an American clinical psychologist, Dr Francine Shapiro, in the 1980s. When a person is involved in a distressing event, they may feel overwhelmed and their brain may be unable to process the information like a normal memory. The distressing memory seems to become frozen on a neurological level. When a person recalls the memory, they can re-experience what they saw, heard, smelt, tasted or felt, and this can be quite intense. EMDR, with its alternating left-right stimulation of the brain with eye movements, sounds or taps during treatment, seems to stimulate the frozen or blocked information processing system.

will be. I travel quite a lot. I take the view 'little and often' for breaks, because I think doing a job of this intensity you need time out."

A final thought from Mark:

Sky's the limit
"There was an occasion when I was asked to do a little piece on Sky News. There had been some government announcement on drugs and they wanted someone to comment, so I agreed. I had to get up quite early and arrived at The Priory at 7am, in my naïve way wondering where the interviewer was, the makeup person, the producer! And there was just a little van and a spotty youth who seemed about 12.

The camera was plonked on the lawn and I had an earpiece. I could hear the producer of Sky News talking over the programme into my ear saying we'll be coming to you soon, just look at the camera. I was getting quite nervous, thinking, 'I could say anything and it would be broadcast live to the nation.' I remember standing on the lawn, feeling a bit of a prat looking at the camera. Just behind the camera a patient, manic and up early, was dancing and prancing and waving at me. I'm trying to keep a straight face as the presenter says '…and now we move to Dr Collins outside The Priory Hospital…', and I'm trying to ignore the patient.

Then things got worse because something went wrong with the satellite, and in the middle of talking to camera my earpiece went dead: silence. So I'm talking to camera and there's nobody there because the chap is in the van and I'm on my own. My kids recorded it and were crying with laughter because I was looking completely gormless wondering what's going on. At last the earpiece came back with the producer saying '…terribly sorry, technical malfunction, we've gone to commercial break, we'll come back to you.'"

See more from Mark in the *Time Out* chapter.

And now for Dr Collins' own gatekeeper…

Lesley Kendrick, Personal Assistant to Dr Mark Collins
Priory years: 1994 – ongoing

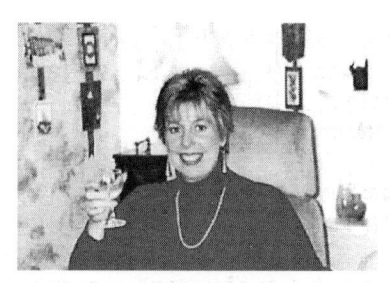

Lesley, at a Christmas Eve gathering

"I was a practice manager at a GP surgery in Richmond and I no longer wanted to save the NHS single-handedly. I was worn out. I thought *I'll have a nice little job in a support role, sit there doing a bit of typing*, and it wouldn't have mattered where it was at the time. That's when I got a job as support secretary at The Priory but after about six months I was spotted by Dr Collins and started working solely for him as his PA.

I remember coming up the drive on my first day and one of the secretaries passing, saying 'You're not coming to work here? It's a dreadful place. I'm on the verge of a nervous breakdown. Nobody cares. I'm leaving.' I thought *Hmm! Am I doing the right thing?!* But I've overcome each obstacle along the way. This place has a very definite pull. Nobody comes here by accident I always think.

Having grown into it over 16 years, there is something fascinating about psychiatry, being connected with people when they're at their most vulnerable. You become part therapist, part secretary, part bookkeeper, and that's what is so good about this job - the variety. It uses each aspect of your personality. There are days when you push the typing away because you think *10 minutes of my time will make a difference to this person.*

The Priory isn't a good place if you're feeling depressed or low because there can be quite negative energies on a bad day. But most of the time, if you're plodding along quite nicely, you just think that could be me and I'm lucky not to be in that position. It helps you count your blessings. It's a bit like Russian roulette. When the phone rings it could be a wrong number or someone standing on Putney Bridge about to jump.

You have to be prepared for the worst and hope for the best. You never know what's coming at you and some days you think, *I can't actually take anymore.* You get awful events, one after the other. On other days people come and say 'Thank you, it made a difference when I was really low and you had time to chat.' That's the reward.

If you do long hours here it does become a large part of your life and you begin to see it as normal, as a little microcosm of the world. Well it isn't: it's a microcosm of the psychiatric world. And I think now and again that gets slightly askew and you need to remind yourself that there is normality out there.

When people realise I work at The Priory, they always ask 'Is there anyone famous in at the moment?' and I reply 'I couldn't possibly say!' Then they might say 'Well I think you'll find that so-and-so was in because I read it in *The Mirror!*' I say, 'I couldn't possibly comment.'

I've found that people open up to you once they know you work in psychiatry. They feel that you're going to understand. You're in a world that's still slightly a bit of a taboo, mental health, however far we've moved on. You realise how many people out there are pretending that everything's perfect but actually they're struggling inside.

The Priory did feel old-fashioned when I first came here, and the technology was a bit behind everywhere else. But in a way I hanker back to that now. As time moves on you realise it had a lot going for it. In another fifteen years, when I'm due to retire, I can imagine thinking, *well, it's probably about time!*"

***

As Lesley describes, there are times when it isn't easy working at The Priory, times when you want to weep, when a particular patient's story touches the very core of your being. But you have to distance yourself. I remember hiring temps who would be reduced to tears when transcribing letters about patients. This might seem endearing but it just isn't practical.

For myself, I lived close enough to make going home for lunch feasible on the odd occasion when it all got too much. Forty-five minutes spent in a quiet place where no one is making demands, relapsing or threatening suicide can rejuvenate the spirit.

Dr Margaret Ballard, Chartered Clinical Psychologist
Priory Years: 1976 – 2000

> When I met up with Margaret in April 2009, she looked back on her years of involvement with The Priory with huge affection.

"The first time I came to The Priory must have been 1976, in the days of Dr Flood. I loved that impressive Strawberry Hill Gothic building and that sweep of rhododendrons. But of course gradually over the years there were more and more sections of lawn which became car park, which spoilt it in my view. But I felt that the environment was very good for patients because it felt like a rather nice country house hotel.

There were two sitting rooms inside the front door – blue was on the right and green was on the left. There were papers and coffee and the sun came in and sometimes the doors were open to the garden. I thought that was lovely.

I had seen people privately at Harley Street but this was my first contact with a private psychiatric hospital. I thought *this is what I'd expect a private psychiatric hospital to be like.* It wasn't until later that I compared it and realised it was better.

I saw patients about every fortnight. If I had two or three patients, I tried to group the appointments together because I was driving out from Chelsea. I continued until a year or two after Dr Kelly left, so in all about 25 years.

During my time there I was asked to do lots of assessments. Sometimes these were for IQ if one of the psychiatrists wondered if a patient's pattern of intelligence might explain their behaviour. Sometimes it was for careers guidance, particularly for people who had been depressed, to find out why their particular job had not worked for them or to redirect them.

There were also patients who it was thought might be dementing, so base line measurements were needed to find out whether a patient's memory and functioning was worse than expected.

Early on I was also involved in monitoring progress in a few patients who had leucotomy operations. I had read about this controversial procedure before becoming involved but these procedures were very much more refined than the original operations made famous in films like *One Flew Over the Cuckoo's Nest*. I assessed patients pre-operatively who were severely obsessional, with psychological tests, some of which were timed. Some could not do the tasks at all or at very slow rates. Assessments took hours to complete. I would re-test post-operatively and found them able to function much more quickly. It did seem to reduce the obsessional symptoms. They speeded up and seemed more normal in their approach to cognitive tasks. I had not believed it would be so effective.

Psychologists are less involved in offering opinions on diagnoses, more often administering tests or offering behavioural therapies. However, I would also contribute to the weekly case presentations, and sometimes provide a second opinion for a diagnosis, for example for psychosis or depression, from my professional perspective.

There was another strand to my work at The Priory, which was behaviour therapy. I ran 8 week sessions for groups of inpatients trying to overcome anxiety problems, phobias and worries. Also I was asked to give lectures, explaining psychological assessment procedures.

Every year there was a Priory Christmas party for both staff and patients. I used to invite my husband James and he really enjoyed them. It was a marvellous inclusive thing to do. As I recall, there was no alcohol (which would have to be so), but there was wonderful food. The chef would be there in his hat, carving the meat. It was a lovely feeling and setting. And you would see patients you had seen before so ill, now functioning.

Perhaps the most important thing in that period was the wonderful nursing staff. You'd go to the ward and there would be a friendly, familiar face. They had the notes and the patient ready. They were very competent, knew their patients and what to look for, and were very supportive to them.

All the doctors were excellent and presented a good team, each with their own areas of special interest. I used to feel that if I ever needed help myself, I would want to go there. The ambience, the nurses, the psychiatrists; I just felt that it was so safe and positive. You would see patients at the beginning of their stay, who were uncommunicative, gloomy, confused, then see them later much improved if not transformed.

I have very fond memories of The Priory. Sometimes when I was leaving, and the rhododendrons were in flower, I'd sneak over and whip a bit off to take home!"

***

Those Christmas parties were a great tradition at the hospital. The long stay patients, in particular, looked forward to them immensely. I noted in 1987, for example, that 300 people attended. These occasions were a marvellous mingling of doctors, patients and their loved ones, and staff. There were no airs and graces; we were all in this together. There might be a string quartet in the mix somewhere and the food was always scrumptious. If a patient felt ill at ease or overwhelmed, they didn't have far to retreat to their room. But the warmth and bonhomie (and close proximity of their protective nurses) made this unusual.

The build up to Christmas lengthened each year, with cards arriving from oversees patients in October. Then the rush was on to shower all the shrinks and staff with gifts. Patients were extremely kind, not only with gifts but with advice. For example, just before Christmas 1992, when I was planning a trip to Wales for the festivities, a delightful outpatient gave me a good tip for travelling alone. She had driven to the far reaches of Scotland one Christmas and worried about breaking down somewhere, stranded and at the mercy of ruthless Scotsmen. So she had a brainwave: she would have someone with her in the car. He would be well-dressed, with a cap worn low over the eyes, and undeniably masculine.

She went to a blow-up doll shop and got one on sale. She dressed him in a tweed jacket, shirt and tie and there was no need to bother with trousers since he had no legs. She figured that when she didn't need him, she would bung him in the boot. Unfortunately, she soon discovered why he was on sale because during the journey he slowly fizzled out through a hole in his groin, until he was just a heap in a jacket and cap. As a friend said later, "What a good job she wasn't caught trying to blow him up again!"

That's a bit naughty, which makes me think of Dr Glyn Davies, a longstanding and very popular Visiting Consultant at The Priory where, in his later years, he ran the Sexual Dysfunction Clinic. I haven't mentioned that. It's a delicate area.

That aside, one Saturday morning I was in the office doing some catching up, when I heard hurried feet coming my way. It was DK and Glyn, tripping over each other to get through the door first. "Glyn has stapled his thumb," DK pronounced breathlessly, "can you phone…". Then as Glyn whimpered behind him, he changed tack: "I must get you to Casualty at Queen Mary's, Glyn", and they jostled to get through the door again. "We can fix that", I cried, brandishing my staple remover, and two sheepish shrinks hurried away.

My role did rather stray into weekends. I remember one Sunday spent reading *The Primal Scream* by Dr Arthur Janov. Dr Kelly was due to meet Dr Janov the following week and wanted me to read and précis the book for him so that he would be able to talk about it intelligently. I sat in Hyde Park for hours, so immersed in the screaming case studies that I felt quite unhinged.

Dr Collins spoke some pages back about the audit the consultants did, that they would take a round of case notes from one of their colleagues and discuss them in the group format. Within the Secretariat, we began our own audit procedure, checking on each other's work as part of our monthly meetings. Inevitably, we would get around to office politics or the introduction of daft new administrative measures. One of our team, Pam, got married relatively late in life, and we were all very pleased for her. It was around that time that she took to catnapping during our meetings. The funny thing was that she seemed to absorb what was going on. I tried it out one day, I said: "What do *you* think Pam?" as the quietly nodded off in the corner. She came to with a start and cried "What do I think? I think it's *outrageous*."

As to my son's earliest days, he learned that he was born at the local hospital, where an early visitor was a social worker; in fact I woke up to find her sitting by my bed. It was assumed that as a single girl I would surely '... want baby adopted'. But when Bob visited, full of macho pride, he insisted that we would be keeping our son and that was that. And when little Robert was chosen for a 'how to bath baby' demonstration, my heart swelled at his flawless performance.

When he was a few months old, Mum went to live in America for a year with my sister, and Bob and I purchased a brand new house and began afresh. Once our home was organised, and having found a delightful baby minder, I got a part-time job as a post office clerk. Bob was not happy about this (he didn't want me meeting people) but we hardly ever saw him anyway, his job taking up more and more of his time. Or so I thought.

It wasn't work. I came home one day to find my personal belongings shoved in the wardrobe, cupboards and drawers; Bob had brought a woman home while we were out and wanted to make it look as if there was no other female around. How he explained the baby paraphernalia was anyone's guess. Perhaps he was posing as a single dad.

In desperation, I answered an advertisement in the post office window. A family needed an *au pair* – 'would accept mother and child', it said. This was our chance.

The lady of the family came round to meet the baby and me and a few days later she and her Land Rover removed the two of us with all our worldly goods. Or nearly all; we had to return days later for our remaining things, when we discovered that a girl had moved in already. Ironically, she was an *au pair*, Swedish.

Once we had recovered from the trauma of leaving his dad and our home, Robert and I were very happy with our new guardians. Their two young boys were great chums for him and their normal family life was balm for our souls.

We would be woken early in the morning by the crowing of the cockerel and the days were a blur of cheeky little boys, household tasks, dogs to walk, horses to be mucked out and fed, chickens to be fed and put to bed and children ditto. I also took on ironing for the family next door, in exchange for riding lessons.

When Bob was (to put it mildly) inconsistent about giving us financial help (I had none of the protection of a married woman), our guardians got a solicitor involved and sought the assistance of the Department of Social Security.

Snippets from the notes the family made at the time highlight how they stood up for us: '...Miss White, although she made the break, only did so because conditions at the home were intolerable with visits by other women and repeated requests to leave,' they documented. 'Technically she did desert the home but only for this reason.'

'...Very shortly after the break, Mr X appeared here to collect the child for an outing, accompanied by a female who had moved into the home. This sort of unnecessarily vulgar behaviour underlines the intolerable nature of the previous arrangements.'

My communication with the Department of Social Security supplied a lighter moment. 'Sometimes, people pretend to be someone else. Does he have any distinguishing features?' asked the DSS officer who would track Bob down. I thought this over and mentioned a varicose vein on his leg. 'Ah', he said dolefully, 'I can't really ask him to roll up his trouser leg, you see. I have to be able to spot the feature at a glance.'

After a while I began to worry about, what next? How long can you be an au pair? What other sort of job would give us a home? The truth was that all I could give Robert was my love, which wouldn't feed and clothe him.

As an unmarried mother at the beginning of the Seventies, I was in a hapless situation. If I had my son adopted, I would be frowned upon for giving up my baby. But if I kept him, I would be selfish for keeping a baby under my circumstances – could I not see the difficulties ahead, and my son's future resentment of our limited, insecure lives?

So the most difficult decision of my life had to be made. I chose the option that guaranteed Robert a future packed with opportunity, security and the love of two parents.

After many emotional conversations with our guardians it was decided that it would be best if I moved to London and they would take care of the adoption. They had seriously considered adopting Robert themselves but realised that I would always know where he was and that the temptation to see him would be too great.

In London there would be no reminders, plenty of work and reasonably-priced bed-sits. The family would interview prospective adoptive parents and ensure that Robert went to a good home.

I quickly found work and a room but the longing for my child was a relentless ache. It felt as if a part of me was missing. My arms were empty and I missed his warmth, his smell, his giggle, and his need of me.

It was winter and my rented room was cold and cheerless. I took long walks in the evenings to get away from the landlord, who was a dirty old man knocking on my door in the early hours. A chair came in handy to jam under the door handle but I felt scared and lonely and overwhelmingly sad. I had one thing to cling to and that was the vision of Robert's new life. I *pictured him, a golden haired boy scampering through fields of happiness, glorious adopted happiness.*

And when he was old enough, he would find me. The waiting had begun.

10
Sleep Your Troubles Away

When he retired from the NHS and St Thomas' Hospital, Dr William Sargant ran a Narcosis Unit at The Priory, admitting all his private patients there until shortly before he died. Narcosis was a controversial deep sleep treatment, for patients who had undergone every other possible treatment without success. Desmond Kelly (Dr Sargant's Houseman in 1959) confessed that when Dr Sargant introduced junior doctors to the treatment, they were frightened silly by the potential risks. But when they saw the results it achieved, they changed their minds.

His methods were certainly controversial. In fact, Dr Sargant (who suffered from depression himself) acknowledged, 'Some say I'm a wonderful doctor. Others, that I'm the work of the devil.' The ultimate pathfinder, his style would not be countenanced today.

Before hearing from the people who worked on the Narcosis Unit, let's have a look at Dr Sargant's life. This man was a huge star in the psychiatric world, so I have indulged in some detail.

Dr William Sargant, Consultant Psychiatrist
Priory Years: 1950s to 1980

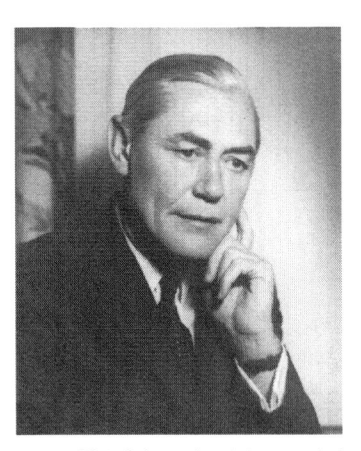

Will Sargant was over 6ft tall, huge in stature and charisma, had the build of a rugby forward and narrowly missed a Cambridge Blue.

William Sargant was born in 1907 to wealthy parents. He was greatly influenced by his father, a staunch Methodist, who instilled in him the need to live a life of service. However, Will couldn't imagine life as a parson and decided on a career in medicine instead. In later years, when he was no longer a believer (despite seeing that religion helped an enormous number of people), he retained the view that 'the true life is spent helping your fellow men.

Will Sargant's rugby skills at Cambridge proved invaluable when his father suddenly lost all his money. The Dean of St Mary's teaching hospital, Lord Moran, stepped in and offered Will a £200 games scholarship. He became rugby captain, as well as playing for the Barbarians, and representing Middlesex.

Yet despite Lord Moran's help, Will's early years at St Mary's were unhappy, with constant anxiety about money. Even when he qualified, financial worries stayed with him because at St Mary's (and all other central London teaching hospitals), it was considered such an honour to work there as a houseman that you weren't paid. For quite a time he lived on "brought in deads", from Hyde Park. St Mary's used to rival St George's on who would do reports on them for the Coroner, and earn a small fee.

Will Sargant rose from being house physician on the medical unit, to house surgeon on the surgical unit. When the Medical Superintendent retired, Will became – aged 24 – the next Medical Superintendent, in charge of admissions, nursing, and junior medical staff. Then a job came up on the Professorial Medical Unit and he began doing research.

This enviable career suddenly tumbled in 1934, when he suffered a severe mental and physical collapse. This was later attributed to pulmonary tuberculosis, which was to affect him again in 1954. Thinking back on that time during an interview in 1987, he said:

> "I was having this terrific career, and suddenly I couldn't do any more. Ten years later, for reasons I forget, I was x-rayed, and there was an enormous calcified region from tuberculosis. So the cause of this sudden collapse became clear, but the fact that no one found it actually saved my bacon, because if I'd had to go and sit in a sanatorium for two years or so, I would probably have completely sunk."

The illness changed the course of Dr Sargant's life. He resigned from St Mary's, gave up rugby and after recuperating at home, secured a six month locum position at Hanwell Mental Hospital in Middlesex (later St Bernard's). Here, at last, he had a nice room and excellent food. In stark contrast, he was horrified by the living conditions of the patients, their suffering, lack of treatment and incarceration. There was only one voluntary patient; the rest were certified and locked in.

The regime was that patients were seen by a doctor every 3 to 5 years. Dr Sargant later described his daily rounds, involving a great bunch of keys, when he would be shown a set of documents, which he had to sign. This meant that the patient was still insane and must be kept there for another appropriate period.

Even in this miserable place there were sparks of humour. Dr Sargant remembered talking to one of the patients during the Hospital Sports Day, who claimed to be the world's greatest bookmaker. 'What happens if you lose money?' Dr Sargant asked. 'Oh I don't do that, because they can't remember what they've backed.'

Will was absolutely thrilled when Professor Edward Mapother, the greatest psychiatrist he had ever met (and who was to become his mentor) invited him to join the staff of the Maudsley Hospital. Will's therapeutic enthusiasm soon became apparent in psychiatric circles. He used amphetamines for treating depression in 1936; insulin treatment for schizophrenia in 1938; and then convulsive therapy (ECT) for severe depression. He helped phase out bromides in favour of barbiturates for sedation, and carried out research on anorexia nervosa and the physiological basis of depression.

In 1938 Will Sargant was awarded a Rockefeller Fellowship at Harvard. During his time in America he enthusiastically furthered the cause of psychosurgery (pre-frontal leucotomy) as a new treatment; indulged in public clashes with supporters of psychoanalysis, and attended parties with his new friends, the Roosevelts.

Returning to England as soon as war was declared, he worked at the Maudsley Hospital's neurosis unit, Sutton Emergency Hospital (later Belmont Hospital), with Dr Eliot Slater. There he saw thousands of acutely disturbed shell-shocked soldiers and with little restriction – which he found a way around anyway when it loomed - tried leucotomies, ECT, acute sedation with 'Pentothal' and 'Amytal', and ether abreactions, with great success.

He saw shell shock at first hand when the hospital took a direct hit from a bomb. One of his colleagues was on the top-floor of the Belmont block when the bomb fell into it and exploded. Dr Sargant recounted, with pleasure, successfully treating him with a half tumbler of gin in the absence of amytal.

Will Sargant wrote the influential book *An Introduction to Physical Methods of Treatment* with Eliot Slater. First published in 1944, it ran to five editions, and Dr Sargant asked Desmond Kelly to assist with the fifth edition in 1972. The work was translated into French, German, Greek, Spanish and Swedish.

He was also the author of *Battle for the Mind,* first published in 1957, and edited by the poet Robert Graves. His autobiography *The Unquiet Mind* followed in 1967. Bertrand Russell said of it, 'every page is of lively interest', and Aldous Huxley referred to '…this very important book.'

In the foreword to his autobiography, Dr Sargant said:

> "The main purpose of this autobiography is to describe the fascinating progress that has taken place during the last 30 years in the discovery of medical and surgical approaches to the treatment of the mind of man. No suffering can compare with the suffering mind or what has been called 'the dark night of the soul'.

I also felt it would interest the reader much more if I wrote this book while my own often unquiet mind was still working at full speed, rather than wait until later when the fire had died down, and one had started to lose that essential feeling for the suffering of one's fellow men, which made the continuous quest described here so very important in my own life."

John Hughes, ex-Chairman & Chief Executive on William Sargant:

"When planning the changes we wanted to make at The Priory, one of my concerns was Dr William Sargant, a towering figure in psychiatry. At that time, aged about 70, he was still hospitalising private patients. I had worked through how we were going to go about remodelling the place, recruiting a couple of new full time consultants, and getting more visiting consultants on board. We had a written business plan but I didn't circulate it because it might seem too radical – hot stuff and embarrassing here and there with respect to old ways of doing things. I made the rounds of all the key consultants to solicit their views, to get acquainted with them, and to try to secure their support for what we were doing.

Will Sargant and I had a conversation two or three months after acquisition of The Priory in September 1980. I took about 10 minutes to lay out what we hoped to do and how it ought to revitalise The Priory, get more patients in, modernise this, do that and the other thing. He was absolutely silent. I had been told all sorts about him, how he was a thundering giant, an overwhelming and towering figure, sometimes belligerent. His tongue could be a two-edged sword, he didn't suffer fools. He could slice people to ribbons and chew them up and spit them out.

I thought that of all the people who might be stroppy and difficult, Dr. Sargant was most likely. So I saved him for last, after speaking with the other key people. I gave him my story and there was a pause. That pause was one of the longest moments of my life, expecting blistering objections. We sat there for I suppose 10 seconds, but it seemed like 10 minutes. And then Sargant said something I shall never forget: 'All that you describe, John, sounds like a very sensible plan. This place is long overdue for major changes. But I give you one warning: the British people and especially doctors are very conservative. When you're sure that you're right about what you want to do, don't let anyone stand in your way'.

I left feeling goose pimples, walking about two feet in the air, thinking that I really hadn't heard that. It was the most supportive statement I'd ever had. And I thought back on that later, over and over again.

I had two pieces of key advice from Sargant. The second one came after he retired and was in his dotage. He and his wife Peggy lived in St. John's Wood. When I was developing Grovelands Priory in 1985/86, I'd often drive right past them on the way to Enfield. On occasion, I'd give them a ring in advance and

> stop in and have a cup of coffee. Once I complained that I had trouble with English Heritage and others over Grovelands. He said, 'John, if you want to convince these people of something, first you must get them *very very* excited!'
>
> He gave me copies of his books *Battle for the Mind*, his autobiography *The Unquiet Mind* and *The Mind Possessed*, the latter all about voodoo, exorcism, and eroticism. He had done one of the most extraordinary and egomaniacal things I've known. He had his autobiography *The Unquiet Mind* published privately as a paperback. He mailed a copy of it to all 1,500 members of The Royal College of Psychiatrists, with a personalised letter.
>
> On the other hand, Will was really quite frail and probably had only a year or so to live, and Desmond Kelly organised a testimonial dinner at The Priory. We had it in one of the big rooms and Kelly and his colleagues of ages past tried to ferret out every single registrar that Sargant had ever had, going back to the 1930s. We had a turnout that filled the room. These people came from all over the world - Cairo, Canada, Australia - it was an amazing thing. Everyone who encountered Dr Sargant in a serious way either loved him or hated him. I was among the Sargant lovers because I found him entirely pragmatic and extremely helpful."

It was during his years at The Priory, when Will Sargant ran the Narcosis Unit, that the family of an Arabian princess he was treating arranged a delivery for him. Gardener Brian Suter recalls the day: "Five different coloured Rolls Royce's came up The Priory drive and parked outside. The first driver got out and asked for Dr Sargant. The doctor came down to reception and the driver asked, "What colour would you like, Sir?" Dr Sargant said "Well, I've always liked the classic black." So the driver handed over the keys, with Sheikh do-da do-da's compliments!"

My own impression of Dr Sargant – and this is despite knowing him only in his later years - can be summed up in the word leonine. His presence in a room was conspicuous, he seemed to command attention.

When Will Sargant died in 1988, one of his old Registrars, David Owen (later to become Foreign Secretary and Minister for Health), wrote to his widow, Peggy:

> "...Your husband was a major influence in my life and I look back on the time I worked for him with immense pleasure. He was the most important figure in post-war psychiatry....All of us if the need arose would have put those nearest and dearest to us in his care – and there is no greater tribute than that. He was a rebel *with* a cause. He understood the awful pain of depression, which drove him to take risks for those who were depressed – because he knew they would take risks with their life. It was a completely different approach to those who could never put themselves in the place of someone depressed."

When Desmond Kelly became a Registrar, Dr Peter Tyrer was the Houseman (later to become Professor of Psychiatry at Imperial College, London and Editor of The British Journal of Psychiatry).

In 2009, Professor Tyrer wrote an invited commentary - *Is research just an optional extra in clinical psychiatry?* - for the Psychiatric Bulletin:

> "...I was present at the eightieth birthday celebrations of Dr William Sargant, head of psychiatry at St Thomas' Hospital, in 1986. My first psychiatric job was with Dr Sargant and he was one of the reasons why I went to St Thomas' Medical School from the University of Cambridge to do my clinical training.
>
> One of the tributes given to Dr Sargant on that occasion was a speech by Professor (subsequently Sir) David Goldberg in which he disclosed a conversation he had had with Professor Aubrey Lewis, the ultimate exemplar of detached scholarliness in academic psychiatry, when he first went to the Maudsley Hospital. When Aubrey Lewis found that David Goldberg had trained as a medical student at St Thomas' Hospital, he asked, amazed, "Tell me something. How does Dr Sargant do it? How has he encouraged so many medical students to go into psychiatry?"
>
> I think I know the answer to this question. Dr Sargant was a charismatic enthusiast who was so far removed from Aubrey Lewis's icy clear-edged thinking they could have come from different planets. He pre-empted Barack Obama's famous three words 'yes we can' when asked if he could treat successfully what appeared then to be intractable mental disorders. "Yes we can indeed. There is nothing we cannot treat, provided the patient is of good previous personality." Nothing could be more exciting to medical students and if a few people were not of good previous personality, what matter. Here was a new discipline emerging from the torpor of therapeutic nihilism to one of hope and optimism and they could get in at the ground floor.
>
> But this is only one half of this story. Dr Sargant was not a first class researcher and he famously criticised Sir Austin Bradford Hill, the inventor of the randomised controlled trial, by claiming that good research could be carried out only 'at the bedside'. What I realised in working with Dr Sargant was that much of what he promulgated constituted hypothesis dressed up as fact. He believed that all drug treatments were better than psychological ones, with the possible exception of Pavlovian conditioning and, like many pioneers in clinical practice, went far beyond his data and his pronouncements on drug treatment. But both Sargants and Lewis' are needed in psychiatry. If we made the best possible combination of the sceptical Aubrey Lewis view of the world with the enthusiastic certainty of the Sargantian approach we would indeed be able to say, 'yes we did.'"

To this day, the Royal College of Surgeons support Dr Sargant's work, saying:

"Although his reputation has declined, his work was of great influence in the biological treatment of depression and the development of antidepressants comes directly from his work."

Sister Eileen MacAuley
Priory Years: 1972 – late Nineties

"I joined The Priory in 1972. One of the things I had to get used to was the grandeur of this place, it was completely different from the big state mental hospitals I had been used to.

I was amazed when Dr Sargant asked me to run the Narcosis Unit. I was young, inexperienced and terribly shy and the great man offered me such a job. I had done psychiatric nursing before but nothing like narcosis. He must have seen some potential in me and I ended up being on the unit for 10 years.

Patients were under narcosis 24 hours a day, except for 3 two-hour breaks for breakfast, lunch and supper. We would wake them at 8am then make them big cooked breakfasts in a sort of walk-in cupboard with a two-ring cooker. They were on massive amounts of medication and it was a case of getting them showered and changed into different bedclothes (they were in bedclothes for 6 to 8 weeks). While they had breakfast we made their beds.

Next we did observations – temperature, pulse, blood pressure – and they had to have a litre of fluids. Then we might give them a wee walk up and down. We had to escort them physically and it was very hard work.

Then we gave them more big doses of medicine – two types of antidepressant, heavy tranquillisers and sleeping tablets. That was back in the days of Mandrax, a very potent hypnotic, which was later withdrawn because drug addicts abused it. Even so, we weren't aware of the controversy surrounding narcosis. I suppose we were young and innocent.

We had to be very careful about observations. Constipation was always a worry because as well as the sleep medicine, they had antidepressant treatment, so it was double trouble. We used enemas when necessary.

The patients treated with narcosis were only those who had been selected because they had been resistant to all other treatments. We had all sorts. I remember patients selling their jewellery to pay for their treatment because they'd been through many other hospitals and nothing had worked. They were people who were seriously mentally ill, with terrible psychotic breakdowns or very resistant depression, and many were suicidal.

But I know it worked. It seemed completely against the grain, against my training, and I wasn't sure I agreed with it. I was trained to motivate people, talk to them, and keep them independent, lively and amused. There were patients that I thought would never ever get better, could not get better. And they did get better.

The average treatment would last six weeks. They also had ECT [electro convulsive therapy], which seems to kick start some chemical that for some reason isn't working.

Lunch at 12 noon, evening meal at 6pm; visitors came at some point in their waking period and we had to have them sitting up ready. Amazingly, they could communicate. It just showed the degree of tension these people had; they could swallow vast amounts of stuff, wake up and talk.

There would be 6 or 8 narcosis patients at a time, some just starting off, and some coming out of it. We had to do everything for them and maybe that's what they liked, all the contact, the protection. There was a real bond between us: they were our babies.

Although at first I wasn't too sure about what I was doing and thought it was weird treatment, later we *believed* in what we were doing. We were there solely for the patient and did everything for that patient's comfort. That is missing in nursing today, that personal touch. People say 'that's not my job, do it yourself'.

In the other parts of the hospital folk were walking about and there seemed to be more cachet somehow. We thought we were up there and forgotten but then we had nobody interfering with us.

Dr Sargant was the inspiration behind narcosis. We knew that 484 patients, who had failed to respond to any other treatment, had been treated with narcosis at the St Thomas' and Belmont Hospitals under his care between 1962 and 1968. The results had been reported in the British Journal of Psychiatry.

I admired this man; I didn't have an affair! I must get this point in. I did *not*! But there was an aura about him. He was a great big Daddy, a gentle giant.

He was distinguished looking but definitely not handsome. He would say to the young doctors or his junior staff 'Make the nurses feel important and they will work for you'. And that's certainly true. There was such trust between all of the staff. He once said to me: 'Don't ever do what you can't. I will always stand behind you in court as long as you are honest.'

Friday afternoons was when Dr Sargant was due on the unit. Everything would have to be ready. Patients would be awake; they wouldn't have been sedated that afternoon. And I was like a queen during his ward round. What I said went (I wonder if what I said was always right?) And he would instruct 'continue treatment', 'stop treatment', 'reduce treatment'. Afterwards, we'd have tea in the office, it was very civilised. The Registrars were in charge when he wasn't there.

To his patients, Dr Sargant was a god. I remember a big company heiress who had nighties delivered from Harrods especially for his visits. And she'd sit there like a model in the bed. And some of the royalty from the Middle East, they adored him. He would sit on the bed beside them and hold their hand; he always had a smile and a twinkle in his eye. It was all done very professionally.

I remember a gorgeous Arabian princess, who arrived with trunks of gear and two slaves with yashmaks. Do you know they literally fed her by hand, not with cutlery, with their hands. I remember the princess saying to Dr Sargant: 'Can I buy you a Rolls Royce today?' And I'm thinking *Yes, and if I could just have a little Mini!*

It was tragic when Dr John Flood died. He'd been here about 25 years and I can't think of anyone that wasn't affected. We felt so much a part of his family. I can remember him coming looking for a razor on the ward. He needed a quick shave and couldn't get into the bathroom at home. We actually felt honoured that he came to us!

When Dr Kelly arrived, I admired his gentleness. He was a caring, quietly spoken man. And very particular, which was good for us because we were kept on our toes. I remember saying to new nurses: 'Be warned: if there's one thing you forget, Dr Kelly will find it. He has the knack of it!'

Eventually the unit closed as there were new treatments available. Some of the drugs became controlled and the local authorities would have been clamping down on it - new anti-psychotics, new antidepressants. But something has to be said for that sort of treatment for those people and how sick they were. I honestly think that all of them got better. Some of them were terribly resistant and took an awfully long time but I can't remember anyone leaving us that hadn't got better.

I then moved to be in charge of the Lower Court ward. It was upgraded and refurbished and that was really exciting because we were involved in the whole process. We had the patients who were too disturbed or too sick to be anywhere else. When you think about the pain and suffering that got them there - and all too often they feel ashamed. If we can make that shame easier, that's what it's all about.

A scary moment was when I removed a gun from under a patient's pillow. I expected to find a bottle of whisky and when I slipped my hand in, there was a gun! I remember running with it wrapped up, all the way to Dr Flood's office.

We protected people who didn't want anybody to know where they were. Maybe we were guilty of reinforcing the stigma but I wasn't going to tell anybody their business. They were very special to me. I'm always proud to talk about my days at The Priory."

Dr Morven Thomson, Registrar and Visiting Consultant
Priory Years: 1976 - 1997

By the time of my get-together with Dr Thomson, at her lovely apartment near The Priory, she was 83. To me, she hadn't changed a bit; still those piercing blue eyes, trim figure and dry Scots humour. In retirement, she enjoys her golf, bridge and grandchildren.

"It would have been mid-Seventies when my boys used to walk along Priory Lane after school. We lived nearby and I would tell them to walk as far as The Priory (I didn't know what The Priory was) and I would pick them up in the car.

This went on for quite some time but when I found out that it was a psychiatric hospital, I decided to investigate the possibility of a job. I was working as a part-time Registrar at Sutton and that's quite a distance, so this idea appealed to me very much.

I walked in one day and spoke to Bridie at reception. 'I'm Dr Thomson,' I said, 'and I'm very interested in working here.' The Medical Director's secretary came down and very shortly I was ushered in to a big office and met John Flood. I had a very pleasant conversation with him. He asked about my experience and said that although he didn't need anyone at the moment, he would remember me.

The fact that he didn't actually ask for my CV meant that I didn't take that too seriously – he was relaxed about our meeting. Some months later I heard that he wanted to see me again. At this point he did ask for a reference. I never got it back. There were these little touches about John Flood. But he did take me on, which was the main thing.

Saeed Islam was already a Registrar so there were the two of us. It was a real plus to find myself working as William Sargant's Registrar. Dr Sargant did modified narcosis at The Priory and only visited once a week so I was responsible for his patients and prescribed their regime.

Sister Eileen MacAuley who ran the unit had a tough time training for the role, until Dr Sargant was completely satisfied. It was a tricky business putting people to sleep like that. The patients had to be fed and to have their excretory functions attended to, and exercised to prevent getting thrombosis. It was difficult - both the nursing and the medical supervision.

Dr Sargant's patients were very ill indeed, suicidal in many cases, manic, uncontrollable. He did something that was very disapproved of at that time: he mixed two kinds of antidepressant, the Monoamine oxidase inhibitors [MAOIs – type of antidepressant] and the Tricyclics [another type of antidepressant]. All the text books said never mix these two but he had no disasters. He had total confidence, so I had total confidence in him.

Nor did he have any hesitation about giving ECT and giving it frequently. Three times a week was standard, but he would give it on consecutive days if a patient wasn't responding. I don't have any memory of his failing with modified narcosis and the mixed antidepressants. In fact he was very successful.

He was a god to his patients and he actually had the appearance of a god (even though he was in his 70s by then) and was the most known figure in the psychiatric world. Controversial, yes, but without any doubt in his own mind that he was doing the right thing. He was an outstanding man.

A lot of nuns and priests were treated at The Priory during Dr Flood's reign. I don't think there was any question about them having to pay. The nuns I treated suffered from depression, and the senior nuns were very much against close relationships between nuns. I learned quite a lot about convents, and I wasn't a bit surprised that so many nuns were patients.

It was some time later that Dr Flood made it known that he was looking for a successor because he was ill, and that he had asked Desmond Kelly, who had said yes. Shortly before John died, I went to his house to see how he was. I was shown into his room and he was lying in bed and one of his beautiful daughters was curled up beside him. He died shortly afterwards.

Then came the day when Desmond Kelly, as the new Medical Director, called a meeting of all staff. It transpired that The Priory had been sold to an American company, CPC, some months previously, without any notification to the staff. John Flood had made this deal without telling Desmond, even though Desmond had of course committed his career to The Priory.

John Hughes's arrival from America gave considerable reassurance – it did to me, anyway. I thought he was a quiet American and quite charming actually! The administration was tightened up and one of the changes was that the nursing staff should wear a uniform. Before that – as in many psychiatric units – they just wore ordinary clothes, the thinking being that patients are panicky, nervous and over-awed, and uniforms don't help. On the other hand, perhaps it's more professional to see a nurse in a uniform – there's a lot to be said for both sides. But it wasn't altogether popular; a soft brown colour was chosen because that suited most complexions.

Dr Kelly turned out to be an excellent Medical Director; he had a different, firmer style. The status of the hospital improved with the establishment of the training rotation of Registrars. That was just one of the positive things he did.

I was a Registrar at The Priory for some years and then applied for a Consultant post at Sutton, where I had been originally. Dr Sargant gave me a very good reference, which of course carried weight. I was appointed and worked at Sutton for 7 years, retiring in 1989 at the age of 63.

I had maintained my association with The Priory as a Visiting Consultant and continued in that capacity for a few more years. The Priory played a large part in my professional life and I remember staff and patients with great affection."

After the initial euphoria of finding each other, there were questions and hurt and anger. My son saw me now, with everything I needed in life, and wanted to know why I couldn't have kept him, why I had rejected him.

We were extremely fortunate to have access to counselling at the Post-Adoption Centre, which helped us, individually and together, to sift through the entangled emotions we were struggling to understand.

Sensing that Rob would soon want to contact his father, I tracked him down via his sister-in-law. She told me that he now lived in Denmark and gave me his contact details. Bob was very emotional when I phoned him and in due course Rob spent a couple of holidays over there. Initially, their reunion was not a huge success, with Rob calling me in high dudgeon. In a subsequent letter to him I said:

> "I know we've talked about the past many times but I think I should now write down a few things. After your telephone call on Thursday, I looked out some notes written by the family we lived with when we left your Dad. They made notes because they wanted to set down the facts. The only reason that the Department of SS and a solicitor had to get involved was because your father was refusing to pay anything towards your upkeep.
>
> Ever since you came back into my life I have tried to shield you from what I really think about your father. That's why at the beginning I said nothing but nice things about him. I think to a certain extent that was the right thing to do because you have decided for yourself what sort of person he is, having spent two holidays with him. From what you tell me he hasn't changed much."

A totally unexpected suggestion made by the Post-Adoption Centre was that I should join a birth mothers group. The very idea that such a thing existed, that I would actually meet other women who had given up their babies, who would understand me because they had been there, was a revelation.

At the meetings, we sat in a circle, maybe 8 or 10 of us, with one or two therapists, and from the very first time I felt totally at ease. These women came from many walks of life, some had gone on to marry and have other children and some had kept their first child a secret. But we shared the sort of heartache that only we could fully comprehend.

One or two had harrowing stories of being sent away to homes run by nuns, where their families hid them for the duration and where they suffered terrible cruelty. One lady, who must have been 65, had been waiting 50 years for her child to find her - I didn't know whether to pity her or applaud her tenacity. Only a couple of us had been reunited with our children.

The Centre also recommended a very good book: *Half a Million Women – mothers who lose their children by adoption*. From the very first sentence – 'Most women who have given up a child for adoption say that it was the most difficult decision they had ever had to make in their lives' – I felt recognised.

11
Last Chance Saloon

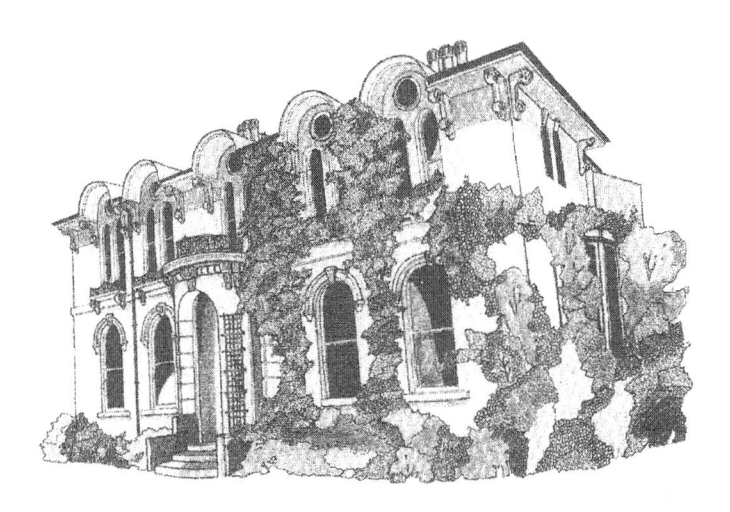

Galsworthy House on Kingston Hill

John Galsworthy (author of *The Forsyte Saga*) was born in 1867 at Galsworthy House on Kingston Hill. The management of the Roehampton Priory purchased the house in 1977 and opened Galsworthy that November as a treatment centre for the growing number of problem drinkers and alcoholics. A mid-Victorian house, it overlooked Richmond Park, with an acre of garden, and was conveniently close to The Priory.

In April 1986, however, the unit was moved to Priory Lodge, within the grounds of The Priory Hospital. Patients stayed at The Priory and underwent detoxification in the main hospital, and attended Priory Lodge (renamed Galsworthy Lodge) for the therapy programme.

The essence of the treatment remained the same – to help patients face the consequences of their addiction and the impact on their families and to learn something of the emotional undercurrents contributing to their dependency. Over the years, the dominance of alcohol as the main substance of dependence has lessened. And now a wide spectrum of dependencies are treated, with some patients being treated for more than one dependency at the same time.

The addiction programme keeps patients busy from 8.30am to 10.30pm and a camaraderie builds up within individual groups, to the extent that many ex-patients make impromptu visits, keep in touch with each other, attend meetings together and provide a distinctly loving and uplifting atmosphere, which is fully evident at the annual garden party.

Dr Max Glatt, Consultant Psychiatrist
Galsworthy / Priory Years: 1977 – 1981

The first Medical Director at Galsworthy was Dr Max Glatt and they could not have captured a bigger name. Dr Glatt always said that he 'drifted' into psychiatry when, as a young German doctor in wartime England, he became convinced that he would be deported when English doctors returned from service. Psychiatry was unpopular and he reckoned that he wouldn't be thrown out so easily if he was a psychiatrist.

As a German Jew, Max Glatt had tried to get out of Germany in 1938 but was caught and imprisoned at Dachau. Then he was deported to England and lived in Kent but when Hitler invaded the lowlands, Dr Glatt was moved to the Isle of Man. Next he was transported to Australia aboard a prison ship. He survived internment in Australia and later came back to England, keen to go back to Germany after the war. When he learned that his parents had died in Belsen, he settled for England.

When Max Glatt first became interested in alcoholism in the Fifties, it was not recognised as a social disease. The government refused to countenance its existence and doctors had no idea what to do with the addicts who came to them for help.

Two decades later, partly thanks to Dr Glatt's work in the field, alcoholism was universally acknowledged as a disease. There were over 30 regional National Health Service alcoholism units, complementing hundreds of Alcoholics Anonymous groups. But that wasn't the end of the problem. Once recognition of the illness was achieved, the political will to treat it withered, the number of units shrank, and during the Eighties more and more costly private clinics opened. Max Glatt became renowned for fighting for help and funding for sufferers, as well as advancing understanding of the illness.

He first came across drinkers while working at Warlingham Park Hospital in Surrey and formed a group of four. Group therapy was in its infancy and Dr Glatt admits that he had little idea of what he was doing. "I asked the group at the end of the hour, 'Has anything come out of this?' They said they had no idea but talking was certainly better than making paper elephants in occupational therapy classes. So we went on." It was clear that something *was* happening. The group's search for its members' salvation continued. They wrote a monthly journal and, once rehabilitated, they arranged annual reunions.

Warlingham Park became the prototype for the treatment of alcoholics within the National Health Service. Until then the government line had been 'What drink problem?' If politicians acknowledged the existence of alcoholics it was only to insist that they could be treated by mental hospitals. The medical establishment was looking at the treatment of alcoholism via the combined Committee for Alcoholics and Vagrants – a title indicative of their perspective.

While stating on the one hand that Alcoholics Anonymous had done more for alcoholics than all the professionals put together, Dr Glatt also said,

> "I come from Nazi Germany, so I have seen what having only one party line can do to you. Anyone can become an alcoholic. It follows that there are very different personalities among them, so to think there's only one method for treating all alcoholics doesn't make sense."

His work at Galsworthy House, later in his career, had to fit in with all the other institutions he was linked with, leading to some erratic time keeping and organisational challenges for Peter Coyle, the General Manager. Despite the frustrations, John Hughes [Chairman & Chief Executive] described Dr Glatt as...

> "...one of these charismatic doctors, a bit like Kelly and Sargant. I suppose I've only met 10 in a lifetime that I would put in that category, out of roughly 2,000. Their critics, who question the outcomes that they publish and the results that they get, can always lay it down to their charismatic treatment, rather than scientific method. And certainly Glatt had that charisma and magnetism - his loyal patients describe him as walking on water. Peter Coyle, too, had that sort of charisma around patients."

John Hughes then recalled more about Peter Coyle, who came in as General Manager of Galsworthy House in May 1977. Just four and a half years later, in December 1981, he died suddenly from a heart attack.

> "He had undergone an earlier bypass operation, but it didn't stop him from chain smoking one cigarette after another. He was a Glaswegian turned West End dandy. Before he quit drinking and turned to a life of helping people recover, he was a manager of cabaret clubs and betting shops for Mecca and Rank. Part of his occupational hazard was that he would go round from club to club every evening in the West End and knock down a couple of drinks in each one. He made no bones about that. He said when he fell off the bar stool that was a great slap. Then he put the same remarkable energy into getting patients better.
>
> Peter was extremely dedicated to the job. I recall his dealing with a titled patient, an earl or duke that we had in custody at Galsworthy House. This chap wanted some special treatment and thought that he should have a bit more waiting on, and that he shouldn't have to do chores (which they did at Galsworthy House). This fellow was a little bit too self-important to do that.
>
> I was present when this issue came to a head and the three of us sat down in Peter's room. The chap was thinking about discharging himself because he was being told what to do and didn't like it. Peter gave the most eloquent speech, in his startling Scots accent, and blistered this fellow up and down. He said 'I don't care if you're a (blankety-blank) duke, everyone falls off the bar stool at the same speed!'

Peter Coyle was an outspoken atheist, and when it came to his funeral, one of his closest pals in the recovery business was Father Tom, a Catholic padre, who was asked to give a non-denominational talk at the funeral. Peter's widow, Sheila, said 'You know Peter wouldn't want you to say anything about God and heaven and hell. What *can* you say?' He said 'Well there are certain things I have to do and certain things I can't do'. They thought about it and then Sheila said, 'Do you have to wear a dog collar because Peter would be upset by that', and Tom said, 'I have to wear my dog collar, but I can put a scarf around it'. It was winter time and the chapel was relatively chilly anyway, so there was nothing terribly out of order for Father Tom to be wrapped up."

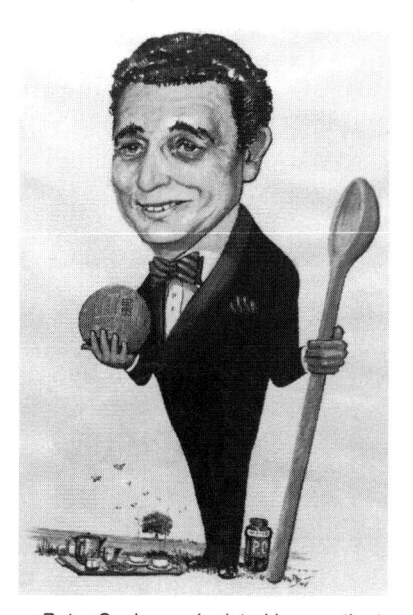

Peter Coyle, as depicted by a patient

When *Outlook* broadcast by the BBC World Service in February 1980 featured a programme on alcoholism, who better to consult than Max Glatt and Peter Coyle. The reporter went along to Galsworthy House to talk about their work and meet some of the patients undergoing the month-long treatment. He discovered that alcoholism is a disease and no respecter of persons. All age groups, all classes are vulnerable, with (for example) journalists, doctors, publicans and company executives particularly at risk. Peter Coyle said:

"There is a big cover up. We think, oh Charlie's quite a lad, isn't he, when he comes back to the office after one of these liquid lunches and keeps everyone alive with these funny stories. But Charlie is ill, very ill indeed, and is going down a slow path which can end in death eventually if it is not checked. But now I am pleased to say that intervention is taking place. British companies are becoming more enlightened. The Americans have been doing this for years. We have been, with typical British reserve, sweeping it under the carpet. And now these companies are actually paying for the treatment. It's usually a confrontation: either you take treatment or you're going to be dismissed."

Dr Rodney Long, General Practitioner
Galsworthy / Priory Years: 1980 – early Nineties

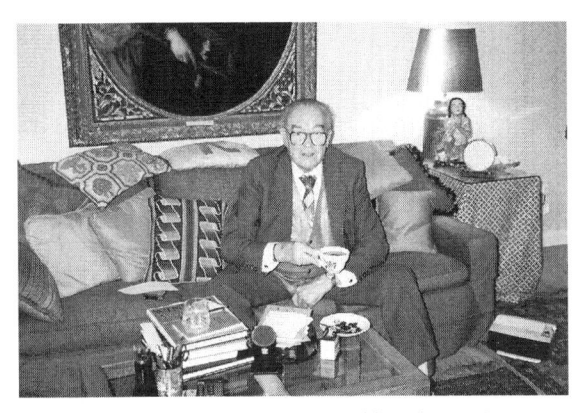

Dr Rodney Long at home during his retirement

Rodney Long graduated as a doctor in 1947 at Guy's Hospital. After doing National Service in the Royal Navy he spent some time in the Merchant Navy and was then Assistant Secretary with the Medical Defence Union, after which he held appointments in psychiatry at Coulsdon Hospital and the Royal Naval Hospital at Haslar.

In 1957 Rodney met Dr Lincoln Williams, a distinguished pioneer in the field of alcoholism. He learnt a great deal from him and took over his practice when he retired in 1963.

Later, Rodney became a General Practitioner in Jermyn Street in London's West End, which probably explains the smart shirts and ties he always wore. By now he had a wide experience of counselling in the field of alcoholism and psychosexual problems. Jermyn Street is a classy part of London so Rodney's patients were top drawer and several famous people sought him out. He was also the medical advisor to local firms such as Rio Tinto Zinc and Walt Disney Productions. Yet he also helped people at the other end of the social spectrum, as Reverend Malcolm Johnson recalls:

> "When I was Rector of St Botolph, Aldgate, I presided over a centre for the homeless, many of whom had a drinking problem. Often in the early days I had no idea what to do so if they showed a willingness to help themselves, I would refer them to Rodney. Of all the people he helped, I remember an educated man in his thirties whom I discovered in a drunken heap on my church steps. I referred him to Rodney who cared for him and healed him. Today that man is a trained social worker, married with two children. He is one of many who will not forget Rodney Long."

Rodney's work at The Priory and at Galsworthy included counselling, group therapy and hypnotherapy, and his methods found great favour with aristocratic patients. He was a very private man – reticent and shy unless he was caring for you as a patient – but once he let you in, he was a very loyal friend. He was funny, too, with many stories to tell, despite suffering from terrible bouts of depression.

Quite by chance, I bumped into Rodney one Friday evening. I had stopped off near Petworth, en-route to Chichester to spend the weekend with my cousin Kenneth and his wife Ann. Running ahead of schedule, I paused at a pub for a glass of wine. Sitting at the bar, I noted that there was only one other customer, a chap who looked rather familiar. It was Rodney (who had moved to Petworth in his semi-retirement) and after that, whenever I went to my cousin's for the weekend I would check whether Rodney was free for a visit.

Rodney had a great collection of old records and would play them whilst recalling episodes from his colourful life. He also gave me tape recordings of his hypnotherapy sessions at Galsworthy House. I still love listening to his terrific BBC voice dipping and soaring as he urges patients to embrace a life of sobriety.

In April 1994, returning from a visit to my sister in the States, I found several phone messages from Rodney. He was at King Edward VII Hospital in Midhurst. I got there as quickly as I could. They had discovered advanced cancer and he died a few days later.

I hope he found his sort of heaven, with music supplied by Noel Coward, Hutch and Elisabeth Welch, beautiful gardens to wander in, a patient or two, and a whisky at day's end.

Rita Murphy, Nurse Counsellor
Galsworthy / Priory Years: 1977 - 2001 and
Graeme Neville-Smith, Sessional Counsellor and Treatment Coordinator *1980 - ongoing*

"**Rita:** I was working for the Inland Revenue in 1977, because it fitted in with my family commitments. But I was keen to get back to nursing and saw a small ad in the *Evening Standard*, which sounded interesting. I was interviewed by Dr Max Glatt, the first Medical Director at Galsworthy, and two weeks later I was working there. I arrived two days before the unit opened, in November 1977.

Graeme: I was Director of the Westminster Advisory Centre on Alcoholism, where Dr Rodney Long was the Medical Consultant. Rodney treated patients at Regents Park Nursing Home. He was a General Practitioner (though most people thought he was a psychiatrist) and he had a practice in Jermyn Street.

Dr Long was approached by Desmond Kelly, to join the Galsworthy team as a Visiting Consultant in early 1980. Dr Long gave my name to Dr Kelly, and following an interview with him, I joined the team as a sessional counsellor in April 1980, mostly involved with groups and workshops at weekends.

It was an exciting time. Galsworthy was one of only three private addiction units in the country, and opened as the field began to grow and assume greater importance in the medical and treatment world.

An important development came about when recovering addicts began to be involved in treatment. It became an essential part of it, but there was always a little division between those who thought it necessary and those who didn't. Later, whereas treatment had been mainly confined to alcohol dependence, more drug addicts were being referred into treatment, particularly when the unit moved to The Priory grounds in April 1986 [to the house that John Flood and later John Hughes had lived in, Priory Lodge].

Rita: When we moved to Priory Lodge, we didn't do any nursing care of the patient, whereas at Galsworthy House, for the last two years, I was the Nursing Director and had a team of 8 staff. But this changed dramatically. I obtained a diploma in Counselling and Consultation, and did a Family Therapy Foundation course, and these gave me more skills for group work. But in some ways I missed that patient contact. Instead, there was a lot of note writing and reports to do, and handovers from the ward staff back to the Lodge staff.

Graeme: It was at that stage that Chris Ball [see later interview] became involved in family work and aftercare and she and I did a lot of work together.

I then took on the role of Treatment Coordinator, interviewing people, and Chris and I used to go out and do a lot of GP surgery visits. That became part of the clinical role.

The AA movement was always very strong, and the programme included regular attendance at meetings nearby, or in the Lodge or The Priory itself. Many people recover through AA, without having any specific treatment. The self-help movement has grown dramatically, with meetings for a wide range of conditions and support – narcotics, cocaine, co-dependence, eating disorders, and families.

Rita: In Galsworthy House days there were one or two quite well-known people and they didn't bring any particular problems such as guards on the gates or newspapers. But when we moved to The Priory grounds, from 1986 onwards, 'celebrity' changed and became quite a difficult problem, with reporters knocking on the door, asking if so-and-so was there. They got short shrift. Patients slept in the main Priory building and walked across the front lawn to Priory Lodge, where the main therapy took place.

Graeme: The staff got a lot of satisfaction in helping others to see that change was possible, provided they didn't drink and maintained a clear head. Also, having the family involved, the aftercare and peer support. I think some staff went home quite worn out by it. There was a great danger of burnout. Being in a closed unit for the day could be quite wearing and highly emotional.

I feel very privileged to share a patient's journey through revelation and acceptance. In recovery you're trying to adopt a new way of life, alter old patterns and habits and bring about emotional change. Quite a task when you have relied so long on a substance for respite.

I've often said to people: the solution is very simple - you need to stop drinking, and with a clear head begin the process of acceptance and change. Of course its more complex than that – invariably a patient comes from a dysfunctional background, has suffered emotional damage, has been subject to trauma, abuse, and neglect. Coming to terms with these issues and being determined to bring about change, achieve emotional stability and perfect a new, less destructive lifestyle is, to say the least, daunting.

Some of us know that even now, years later, social occasions are still a bit uncomfortable because we're probably in fact quite shy, maybe suffer social phobia, perhaps don't like people all that much, a little bit suspicious still. So getting in there and being part of it is not easy, when the way you've done it before was to use something to arm yourself before even starting. That's the difference.

Rita: I got much satisfaction working with families, the aftercare groups, patient and family groups, seeing the patients coming back, doing well, talking about their recovery. I found the most headaches came from patients who started drinking or using drugs when in treatment. That was very disruptive within the group. Also, patients who rebelled against the unit's boundaries and rules.

Graeme: The advantage of moving to The Priory grounds in 1986 was that we were closer to the main body of referring consultants. Dr Craggs was the Lead Consultant with responsibility for the Lodge, and under his guidance there was greater involvement on all sides – consultants, nursing staff, and management. Not everyone thought that was a positive move but in fact we began to get more referrals from all the consultants.

Rita: It's difficult to put into words what it felt like to be in a particularly productive group session or one-to-one. You came out with a good feeling that there had been a breakthrough. The ex-patients garden parties would give you a buzz. We'd talk about it for the next day or two – who we'd met, how well they were doing.

I can remember a couple of incidents when things went a bit wrong. We had a resident chef on Kingston Hill, I'll call him Hank. He was known to be a very hot tempered man in the kitchen. Galsworthy was hosting a conference for GPs and Consultants one day and guest speakers were invited and an impressive lunch was to be provided at the end of the event. Imagine the embarrassment and dismay of the Galsworthy staff when in the middle of the presentation, in the kitchen next door, plates were being hurled, Hank was coming out with expletives, and his kitchen hands were in floods of tears. Fortunately, Peter Coyle was there to deal with it. We laughed afterwards and I think the doctors who heard the commotion saw the funny side of it but it wasn't funny at the time.

We had another resident chef, who had a room on the first floor. He had an additional door in his bedroom which when open looked down on to a toilet below. It was probably an area that hadn't been finished off when they were converting the old building. Anyway, it was handy for him because it meant that he didn't have to walk downstairs to pee. But it did require good aim. One day nature called and he flung the door open in full readiness and who was more surprised, the patient sitting on the loo or the young chef poised and ready to fire?! It caused a lot of merriment, and fortunately the patient concerned had a very good sense of humour.

Graeme: Remember the patient in his pyjamas who went over the back wall into Richmond Park? He was in search of a drink. That caused a bit of a stir.

Rita: We often had to run down Kingston Hill after patients and find them in the pub at the bottom of the hill. When I think about it, most of my fond memories are of Galsworthy House, on the hill.

Graeme: It was intimate, a very close environment, and part of it was the pioneering thing too. The other Priory hospitals hadn't started up yet so it was a bit of a forerunner."

Dermot, Patient & Painter/Decorator
Galsworthy / Priory Years: 1985 - 2006

> When I interviewed Dermot, we met at Brian's home (ex-Priory gardener). Brian features in *Maintaining the Fabric* but couldn't resist chipping in with Dermot.

"**Dermot:** I became an inmate at Galsworthy House on Kingston Hill. Basically, I had a very slight drink problem. I went to see my Mum's doctor, who was private, and he said come up and have an interview at Galsworthy (which I don't remember) and I woke up there the next day. I didn't know where I was. I thought I must have booked myself into a hotel, and went round looking for the swimming pool. I was shocked to find that I was in a bloody bin! July 23rd 1985.

But being with a bunch of other people who had a problem with drinking, being with other alcoholics – I suppose I'd found my tribe. After a week I was taken to an AA meeting: I did not want to go to an AA meeting. I'd heard of them but whatever they were, I didn't fancy them, they sounded scary. But I was given a choice, as everyone is: if you don't go to AA, you leave. It was the rigorous 12-step approach.

So I went to a meeting. I was horrified that people were talking about things which I thought should be kept secret at all cost. They were talking about feelings: imagine saying that you're afraid! I went to different meetings, such as Pont Street, that was a big one, very intimidating at first, maybe 100 people. You wouldn't share or even open your mouth there. When I left Galsworthy I carried on going to meetings.

I was at Galsworthy for about 5 weeks, and when I left, they said, 'What are you going to do?' I said, 'I haven't got a bloody clue.' 'Why don't you come and work for us? You could look after the building; do whatever needs to be done.' I thought *why not? I'll be talking to patients all day, if I want to.* So I did. And then as a voluntary thing, I bussed patients out to meetings and that carried on when we moved to The Priory grounds. Quite a few ex-patients did that.

When Galsworthy on Kingston Hill closed in 1986, most people were made redundant. John Hughes got in contact with me and said 'I gather you're going into business for yourself as a builder and decorator. Give me a price for painting the offices at the Lodge.' I gave him a price and he said 'Right, come along and do it.'

From then on, for about three months of the year, I worked in The Priory building itself, with a small team. What a lovely old building, and that antiquated basement with the huge flagstones. Initially, I worked for John Hughes and then Erich Herrmann started using me. That's when I got to know everyone at The Priory. I didn't tell anybody my background; I didn't want to break my anonymity.

We worked to a high standard, using traditional methods of restoring. I was probably far too cheap, that's maybe why Erich used me! But it was very good for me. Say if something had to be done at night over at the Eating Disorders Unit, I could finish and go to an AA meeting right there, either in the chapel or across at the Lodge [on the other side of the lawn].

I remember a very intelligent lady patient, and somehow I didn't expect this from her. I was on one of the wards, fiddling with an electric socket by a door. She came up and said 'Have you painted that door?' I said 'Yes, previously.' She said 'I don't like that colour,' bashed me on the head, and walked off! You do have to be careful at The Priory.

Brian: Then there was the time that same patient was screaming down the hallway to Dr Kelly. I was at the nurse's station with some of the nurses, and the patient was quite high this particular day. She had been waiting for Dr Kelly and she spotted him going into another patient's room at the end of the corridor. She screamed at the top of her voice: 'Desmond, you old queer, when are you coming to see me?' At which point everyone wanted to dive into a hole. He marched down to her and said 'Now you know I'm not gay, I've got a wife and two children.' That was her way of getting his attention!

Dermot: There was another patient who was permanently there, always went around in a suit. For the first six months I worked there, I actually thought he was a doctor. But he was mad as a hatter.

Brian: He was always waiting for a phone call from MI5; always waiting to hear from 'Z'! He – let's call him 'N' – called Erich into his room one day and said, 'Have you heard?' Erich said, 'Have I heard what?' He said 'The Hospital Director's gone. What do you think?' Erich said 'I thought he was quite a nice chap, shame for him to go.' 'No,' said N. 'Me! What about me taking the job? I could do it.' That night, N was sectioned [under the Mental Health Act]."

> I chipped in myself here, reminding Dermot that he and I share an interest in the hospital's history. When he had shown me some old ledgers that he had retrieved from a skip, I was horrified that they had so nearly been dumped. Another time, Brian brought me some photos dating from the 1870s. He had found them in an outhouse somewhere in the grounds. He had put them in his wheelbarrow and had been told that they should be thrown away too. I must admit that this knowledge still fills me with impotent fury! We saved some ledgers and photos but inevitably others were lost. Here's what Dermot said on the subject:

"**Dermot:** In about 1994, I was going outside the back door to the car park and there was a skip there and inside were all these brown leather-bound ledgers, books and papers, all bundled up. They filled about half the skip. You touched them and your hands came away brown. I took one out and opened it and it contained all the nursing records of patients from the 1870s, beautifully handwritten, with Dr William Wood's notes in the margins. There were folders with patients papers, death certificates, everything. In that skip was the whole history of psychiatry at The Priory; part of the country's medical history.

I got some of them out. I think I asked Erich, what's happening with this stuff? He said the skip was going the following morning and it was all rubbish. Anyway, some were saved.

I did have a look through one or two of the books but I found it very hard to read all that slanted longhand. But I became convinced that Jack the Ripper had been at The Priory: the dates of a particular patient were spot on and he used to leave the place at night. So I am the only person who really knows who Jack the Ripper was!

I've made some wonderful friends through Galsworthy and The Priory. But the last thing I had been planning to do was give up drinking. As far as I was concerned, drink was the solution to everything."

This next anecdote from Dermot is a peach:

From one AA to another

"There was an incident around 1987 time. We were working at night, painting and decorating. I had 2 or 3 people working for me and another person, Mike, came along to give me a hand. I'd met him in AA - he'd been in treatment too, but not at The Priory, and he was getting re-established. He was an actor and sometime director, but he was resting between gigs, you could say. He was driving a 3-ton lorry and had to start his own work at 6am.

Anyway, he came to help and we did the work then went across to an AA meeting at the Lodge. We came out, full of spirituality and the joy of living, went round the back of The Priory to the car park, and saw that all Mike's tyres were flat. We thought someone must have climbed over the wall and slashed them. But we looked again and the tyres hadn't been punctured. We went to reception and they said, 'Oh yes, they have all been let down.' We said 'Why? Why are you letting tyres down? Could you please tell us? We're in shock here.'

Mike was getting a little bit distressed by then. They told us that Dr Kelly had given orders for them to be let down because he didn't know whose lorry it was and people had been parking there illegally. He thought this lorry must be owned by thieves who later in the evening were going to load it up with all The Priory treasures and disappear.

That's when Mike lost it. 'Is this doctor a fucking patient? What's his name, Kelly? He should be in a fucking straitjacket!'

I don't think Dr Kelly would actually do it himself but he'd asked someone else to do it, and we didn't have security then. Finally, we got AA (the Automobile Association, that is), and they thought it was quite funny.

Then another AA man had to come along because they didn't have the right jack for a 3-ton lorry. The AA had to take every wheel off and take them to the garage. It took 2 or 3 hours.

In the end, the lorry was back in running order and Mike had calmed down a bit. But still, I think if Dr Kelly had walked round the corner he might have left on a stretcher. Then Mike said the immortal words: 'That man has set my recovery back five years.' I know Dr Kelly still feels guilty about it. And so he should! He asked me what Mike was doing now. I said he was up North, directing in the theatre."

***

As his loyal ex-P.A., I must add here that the tyres operation *was* carried out by Dr Kelly himself, together with the Deputy Hospital Director at the time. DK would not expect others to target suspicious vehicles if he wasn't prepared to do it himself! There had been a spate of audacious burglaries, including the snatching of televisions when patients were actually watching them.

Chris Ball, Programme Director
Galsworthy / Priory Years: 1984 – 2005

> Chris Ball and her husband Richard Steele now split their time between Portugal and England. We met up all too briefly in Portugal. She is great company and a wonderfully intuitive therapist. We recalled being on one of the outward bound management courses together. I was rooming with Chris and another expert in addictions, and before nodding off I would listen to them talk business. "The thing that must put some people off going through your programme or going to AA," I butted in, "is the constant reference to God." And Chris said a very good thing: "Then don't think of it as God, think of it as Good Orderly Direction." I liked that. Chris has taken up golf, which has become "...a totally positive addiction!"

"The addiction unit was originally a private clinic, Galsworthy House, on Kingston Hill. I went to enquire if there were any patients who would like some extra help. I was working with the Westminster Counselling Service, running a little office in Tolworth near Kingston. They suggested instead that I apply for a job they would be advertising the following week. It was a new post, as Case Manager, and the idea was (where appropriate) to encourage enquirers into having treatment, which was to be 4-6 weeks as an inpatient. The interview was at Galsworthy House and I was told I had the job straight away! My most important task was to let people who otherwise would have been lost in their addiction, know that there was hope for a seemingly hopeless case. Another task was to make Galsworthy treatment a household name. Of course it then became The Priory and it *is* a household name.

I was familiar with the 12-step programme but I had been at drama school and in the theatre, and done a degree in Drama and English. Then it was suggested that I do Drama Therapy, so I was passionate about Drama Therapy and about the 12-steps when I went to Galsworthy. And the AA programme is all about the 12-steps.

My role evolved as I developed new ways to spread the word. For example, we gave presentations at GP surgeries and took packed lunches for them, otherwise they wouldn't have had time to listen. It had to be appealing so the packed lunch had to be exciting – wine, beautiful sandwiches. They were interested because they were eating.

For the next two years it was just me answering all the enquiries that came into the clinic, and that was when I met Desmond Kelly. He was always eager to back what we were doing in the addiction unit. So much so, that he invited me to set up a little group at The Priory Hospital itself, to see if I could entice some of his patients – the ones with a suspected alcohol problem – to simply begin talking about their drinking habits. This was very exciting and they were great little groups, often successful in that a patient would agree to come into the addiction unit and do something about their drinking.

Things changed when I was called to Head Office one morning to see the Chief Executive, John Hughes. He told me that we were closing down Galsworthy on Kingston Hill that very day and moving to the Lodge, in the grounds of The Priory Hospital. The move had to be carried out very responsibly because the patients, when they knew they were moving, were a bit hysterical. I had no idea this was going to happen.

I would be running this new unit and was told I could select two staff members to stay on. One of these was Rita Murphy, a nurse who became a Nurse Counsellor and one of the backbones of the Lodge addiction unit. She was very important to us, very stable and sound.

Dr Craggs was the Medical Director of the unit. He was direct, no nonsense, practical. He and Desmond Kelly were our biggest allies. It was a professional programme, anchored by a strong and supportive directorate in Dr Kelly, Dr Craggs, and a supportive team of therapists.

So we started all over again in the new building and I had to run the groups, timetable and new staff (which weren't many). I think the move was an incredible improvement. We retained patients more easily – they used to discharge themselves quite often at the other unit but I think they felt differently now. They had to go into the main building to sleep and walk across the lawns to the Lodge. I think it felt like they were going to school for the day, and was much less threatening. They stayed at the Lodge for the day, had lunch there, and went back in the evening.

I always thought it was fair enough that people had to pay for addiction treatment because otherwise there was nothing. Governments have never offered good addiction units like The Priory; if they had, The Priory wouldn't have existed. Well actually they did, there were a couple in my early days, but they closed them down. St Bernard's was a great one but it was a rough old place and you had to be tough to get through it.

I'm not a technician. You can teach me all you like about being a therapist and it will go in one ear and out the other because I'm not very bright at that. I just work with where we're at. I remember one girl who came in, she used to crouch behind the cooker in the kitchen and hide. So I would go into the kitchen and get my coffee and talk to her! She wrote to me about four years later to say 'thank you for treating me as normal, when I was crouching behind the cooker!'

What I loved about the Lodge was that we didn't have too much talking – we didn't have lectures. We had drama therapy and groups, when we worked on what was happening here and now. And things like intimacy - there's an exercise where you take off your shoes and socks and sit with a partner and massage each other's feet with your foot.

One of the things in groups I was also passionate about was going for that 'empty space'. For example, if I'm sitting with you for five minutes and we don't speak, we'll get uncomfortable. Now if you're an addict you really feel you have to fill that space because you feel inadequate just to sit there. You don't know what the other person is thinking about you, so your self-criticism comes in. And to go into groups, which have 25 people sitting around, and to be left with that space when the group is focused on you... And I say, for instance, 'can you say that without speaking?' And the person is left without all the tools they think they need to have. So it's incredibly exciting, much better than stating: 'you're angry!' Where does that get you?

Also, I think people have to find their own way, and that was part of the success of the Lodge. I think at first, as a therapist, patients hate you because they think you're going for them. But you're not actually, you're just letting them find their own way, so they can get past hating you and thinking you're making fun of them or something. It is really important that you don't do the work for them.

People do radio and television programmes about addiction units and they always go to the patients. I always thought they should do a programme that goes into the staff room because if you listen in the staff room, you hear everything about addiction and everything about patients.

Well-known clients were no more or less difficult to handle than anyone else. And I don't think it was unusual that some of the celebrities were so helpful; everyone wanted to do their best for the cause when they became well.

Eric Clapton was a big part of the Lodge. He was my husband's friend to start with and then I met him. Later, he wanted to talk to me about going through a bad relationship so we did talk and he used to come to The Priory. Then he rang one day and said, 'I just want a hug and a cup of tea,' and came in and just started talking to people. He trained on our peer supporter course then came and did groups. And he got paid. He loved the thing of being paid.

Eric was magic. We used to run groups together and his timing (groups are all about timing) was fantastic. Now he's got Crossroads, his own addiction unit in Antigua and it's doing really well. That's what came out of Priory Lodge; he wanted Crossroads to be modelled exactly on the Lodge. He talks about it in his autobiography *[Eric Clapton The Autobiography]*.

Camaraderie was always the purpose of our treatment programme; it was for people who weren't connecting. Addicts wouldn't be addicts if they could connect."

Alex, a patient

"Severe depression took me to The Priory. I saw my GP and admitted that I was depressed again. She asked me whether I could be an alcoholic. Being such a people pleaser I did the drinks diary and she asked me to go to

Alcoholics Anonymous. I went to AA and cried my eyes out and realised something was seriously wrong. Of course when I stopped drinking, I went completely barmy because I had been self-medicating with alcohol and no longer had an emotional crutch.

A lovely lady took me under her wing, an ex-Priory patient. She said, 'I think you ought to go and see a psychiatrist.' I always knew at the back of my mind that there was something wrong but I had always thought that if I ended up in a loony bin or a prison I would commit suicide.

There was no treatment available within the NHS. I went to The Priory and had a look around beforehand, just to see what type of people went in, and with no intention of admission. The staff were brilliant and treated me with enormous dignity, taking away my shame of being mentally ill. I agreed to do the Galsworthy rehab programme and three days later I packed my tennis racquet, swimming costume and my own pillow. I drove myself and put my pushbike in the car. I knew they confiscated car keys. My back-up plan was to leave the car unlocked so I could escape on my bike.

I met a woman making tea in the kitchen and she told me it was the best thing she had ever done, coming into The Priory. She was really kind but I thought *Best thing she's ever done? How sad.* But it turned out to be the best thing for me too.

I knew they locked everyone out of the bedrooms during the day so I presumed you could lock yourself in at night – incorrect. Having post-traumatic stress disorder, the first night I built a little barricade and set up an alarm system using the metal wastepaper bin.

At the beginning of rehab I was put into *baby* group as a new girl. There were six of us and each time there was a break, the other five went out for a fag. I had never smoked before but within a week I was smoking Benson and Hedges. It was all so intense and emotional. I was petrified that I was going to have a nervous breakdown, because I always felt on the edge. I remember a lecture on why and what alcoholics drink on – for example, envy. Then there was lust. Being a bit of a traumatised rape survivor I said '*Lust*?! Fuck that!'

The counsellors had seen all types and knew the mind of an addict – I soon discovered that my methods of survival – charm, manipulation, persuasion, and personality – weren't working. I was made the scapegoat of the patient group because I was provocative, rebellious and anti-everyone. I think the first thing Dr Collins heard of me was about a girl who had thrown a lemon meringue pie at the wall in the garden. My mother always used to make meringue pie for my brother. I was out of control, scared, and depressed.

One night I ran away and hid in the chapel. There's a lovely antique sideboard in there (my degree is in antiques) and I lay underneath it and tapped in to the 19th Century carpenter who made it. I could hear everyone shouting for me.

When I got a bollocking, I said 'Well, it's a spiritual programme – why didn't anyone look in the bloody chapel?'

Another time I ran away from an AA meeting which we were bussed out to. I didn't go far. I met someone in the AA group, an ex-patient, and she said 'Look, I think you're going to have to ring up and turn yourself in.' So I got a taxi back and they breathalysed me and sent me to bed.

My group did a petition, complaining about the food and about their bed sheets – 'this place costs more than the Ritz'. There were two actors, one very famous, and he was leading this petition of complaint. I'm not frightened of being controversial nor star-struck and I refused to sign it, which made me unpopular again. I said, 'If you want new bed linen, you just go to the fucking cupboard!' Being an over-eater, I loved all the food. I wrote a letter to the chef saying, 'you're going to get a letter of complaint but I just want to say that your food is absolutely fantastic.' That letter ended up in my medical file.

I ran out of group one time and Chris Ball came after me and we sat on a bench. She said, 'Are you aware of how much attention you need?' I thought, *oh my God*. It was like being back at school but she was right and I've mostly grown out of that now. Arguments and displays of emotion ran high. I look back and smile at a huge row I had with an actor. I had crept into his room and put my cuddly Pink Bunny next to his teddy bear to show my support. He was insane with fury at me for invading his space. It was a tricky environment and I felt I could do no right.

The nurturing and love came from many unexpected staff members such as Clara the cleaner, Bobby from maintenance, Dr Mark Collins and his wonderful secretary Lesley Kendrick, and ward nurses. The counsellors did a fantastic job but I never felt nurtured. A night nurse, Irish Tony, used to say 'If you're going to have a breakdown, can you do it in the morning? Can you just wait until the day staff?!'

It was an inner battle because I knew the insurance would only pay once: I had to stay. That triggered all sorts of things. I got reprimanded for playing tennis in the middle of busy Priory Lane to get run over. Later I played against a wall safely inside the car park using crockery as a ball. The sharp crockery cut my racquet strings, so that was the end of that.

I cried every day for three weeks and either people gave me a wide berth or accepted me weeping for hours and hours. At the end of the third week I was asked to look after a new patient who had just arrived. I was amazed. I couldn't understand why they had asked. Of course I do know today – recovery is about helping others too. I was introduced to Welsh Claire and we clicked immediately. She made me laugh and from then on laughter and love became my saviours. We acted like two naughty schoolgirls and the element of fun came back into my life. By the sixth week I was actually voted in as Deputy Group Leader by the group – miracles of recovery commenced and still continue today.

You go in for one thing then they label you with more. At the 10 o'clock group at night, the addictions got more and more. I first go in and say 'I'm an alcoholic.' About week two, it was, 'I'm an alcoholic and an addict pill popper' (because I never took drugs, I only took over the counter pills so that I could feel I wasn't an addict). Then over-eating: so I was an alcoholic, an addict pill-popper and an over-eater. Then I became a smoker. I hate smoking! But I gave that up a few years later. I ended up having a triple diagnosis – addiction, bipolar disorder and post-traumatic stress disorder.

When I wasn't getting on with the group, and in the days when you could sit anywhere in the dining room, I sat with other patients. I spoke to one guy and said 'What do you do?' He said 'I'm a consultant here.' Next day he was a nuclear scientist. On the third day he was a concert pianist.

The first stay at The Priory (which I call the savage visit) was when I was mentally and spiritually ripped to pieces. Physically, I was made to do yoga and tai chi on the lawn. It made me really angry. I suppose, like the rape, I was being forced to do something physical that I didn't want to do. I lay rigid on my mat and refused to move. I did, however, like walking around Richmond Park and feeding the ducks – interaction with ducks I could cope with. Once a week we were marched next door to the Bank of England sports club."

Alex completed the Galsworthy programme and was also referred to Dr Mark Collins for Eye Movement Desensitisation and Reprocessing (EMDR).

"EMDR was quite innovative in 1999. I actually had it at the same time as Galsworthy, so I went completely nuts. I don't think they do it at the same time now because it can be so severe, and now they have light machines and all sorts of things. But in those days Dr Collins did it with two fingers: Dr Wriggly Fingers.

I was very eager to do it. One of the first times, I broke down in tears, absolute hysteria. Another time, it was a cellular memory, I was being strangled. I remember him saying, 'This has happened before and you didn't die. This is just a memory.' It was so physical – rendered me shaking for 24 hours."

I asked Alex to explain EMDR to me…

"Let's say that today you ran over a cat and you were a bit traumatised. You go to bed and you have rapid eye movements. It's as if there is a filing clerk sitting in the back of your mind. He comes rushing to the front and says 'ok, run over cat, let's file that in the memory bank'. The following day you're still a bit traumatised but you're not as bad because he's filed it in the back. Within a month it goes into the archives. The problem with post-traumatic stress disorder, my memory was never filed and my mind remained on red alert, almost as if it was happening. EMDR simulates rapid eye movement and that gets the filing clerk into business.

Eighteen months later, I went back for more EMDR. It was so severe and harrowing that I ended up being there for 5 weeks. I only went in for a night. I was 18 months sober but it was so disappointing because I still felt suicidal. This I called my 'namby-pamby' visit – no strict rules and fellow angry patients in withdrawal ready to pick on anyone. Art therapy every day with another fellow alcoholic in recovery. The non-addict inpatients were nicknamed the *glums* and we were the *wineglums*. I remember one poor glum young man with his arm in plaster having thrown himself out of a window the week before. The glums would be doing their art therapy very slowly but not us. The art therapist said 'Can't you two just slow down a bit?' We said, 'Why?'

As to my Bipolar Disorder (manic depression), that wasn't diagnosed until I streaked across The Priory lawn at night! During the day I was feeling extremely low. By night-time I had organised a sponsored streak in aid of a children's cancer charity, which I considered to be quite sane. The staff thought differently and thankfully I had a diagnosis and medication which changed my life.

During one EMDR session, I said 'I feel like Edam cheese; like my heart is covered in red wax, stopping any love going out and love coming in, stopping a flow of positive energy.'

A bit more treatment and Dr Collins said 'what can you see now?' At the top I could see a bit of yellow coming through, it was thinner at the top and thicker at the bottom. Then it came down to half way and the heart became a woman. I said 'Oh, she won't drop her trousers' (it was all to do with rape). He said, 'What would be good would be a fig leaf just there on the heart.' Then all the wax melted away and it was just a yellow heart with a fig leaf on it. And that was the one I drew in art therapy.

As I got better, I was so touched by the compassion and professional, continuing care I had received that two years later, when I went on a retreat in Greece, I said a little prayer: what can I do to give back? Bang out of nowhere the idea came, to create a fund. So began my charity, the Yellow Heart Trust, and Dr Mark Collins is our Patron.

The charity was born in his office. It has been a lot of hard work and tears. We are at the point now where the charity is a teenager. It was my baby and I have to move it on. One of the things that can stop charities is the founder.

My friend who is a survivor of the Marchioness [the pleasure boat that sank after colliding with a dredger on the River Thames in August 1989], Philip Robinson, wants to take it over. I will still be part of it but will take a step back.

When I received a letter from 10 Downing Street saying, would you accept an MBE, I obviously thought it was a scam. I shoved it in my pocket and showed it to a friend later. I said 'Do you think this is real?' 'Of course it's bloody real!' It was for 'Outstanding Service to Disadvantaged Women by founding The Yellow Heart Trust'.

My parents were so proud, after all those terrible school reports they had to endure. When I'm feeling low, when everything is going wrong, I think well, I can't be that bad. It's one of the things that keep me going when I'm depressed actually.

Even today, I would love a glass of champagne; I'll always want to drink. My fantasy was that if I ended up in a nursing home I'd be the old dear with the vodka. But someone said, 'When you're in a nursing home, Alex, they will have complete control over you.' That ruined my fantasy. But I think when you die you get up to the pearly gates and you see Saint Peter. He hands you a glass of champagne and he says 'Alex, all you need is the one and it will be bliss. So come on in.'

Being an addict, what I have achieved for the Yellow Heart Trust is not enough. It's never enough. But I'm glad I fulfilled what I vowed to do."

***

As Chris Ball, the Programme Director said earlier, she got to know Eric Clapton through her husband Richard. In his book *Eric Clapton The Autobiography* he describes how, whilst entertaining Chris and Richard in Antigua, he confided in her about a relationship.

> "She looked at me as if I had landed from another planet. 'Why are you giving this woman all your power?' she asked. I had no idea what she was talking about, but I was intrigued. Chris was at that time director of the alcohol and addiction unit of the Priory psychiatric clinic in Roehampton, but I had heard that she also conducted one-to-one private counselling sessions. I asked if she would see me, and she said yes. For a while, I didn't really know what I was getting into…"
>
> Chris' first question to me, at our very first session was, 'Tell me who you are,' a very simple question you would think, but I felt the blood rush up to my face, and I wanted to yell at her, 'How dare you, don't you know who I am?' Of course I had no idea who I was, and I was ashamed to admit it. I wanted to appear that I was ten years sober, and fully mature, when in fact I was only ten years old, emotionally speaking, and starting from scratch."
>
> …I began doing peer-support work at the Priory, which involved taking a short training course, and among other things allowed us to sit in on group therapy sessions with clients at the beginning of their day. I loved it, it gave me a sense of real responsibility, and at times it was like living theatre; you never knew what would happen next, and the results could be so positive, sometimes miraculous."

***

One lunch time I had to go over to Galsworthy to check something with Chris but she was just about to go into a meeting with some of the Galsworthy team. "Why not join us?" she asked, "they all know you and you could find it interesting." So I sat and observed the therapists supporting each other and discussing their own thoughts and issues. I even took part. Then who should join the gathering but Eric Clapton, who had been doing some peer support work. To say that he participated fully would be a huge understatement. He positively oozed enthusiasm for their combined task of helping others. He described the reciprocal support of the team as better than any other high he had known.

***

In his autobiography *Gazza My Story*, football legend Paul Gascoigne relates how he was to experience Eric Clapton's peer support in 1998. But first he explains how Bryan Robson [Middlesbrough Manager] ...

> "...dragged me into his car and we drove off. The next thing I remember was arriving at a big white building. It was the Priory, in south-west London – one of the country's leading private psychiatric hospitals, famous for treating celebrities for eating disorders, alcoholism and drug abuse, among other things – though I didn't know that till several days later.
>
> They knocked me out for about four days, gave me tablets, tried to detox me. When I returned to some level of consciousness, they put me on a twenty-four-hour watch, fearing I might still be suicidal, that I might jump out of the window. I still didn't know what was going on, or quite where I was, or why. When I eventually sobered up, I asked what was happening. It was then that I was told I was in the Priory, suffering from alcoholism and depression, and that they were going to make me better."

After a few days when he just stayed in his room -

> "...there was a loud knock on my door, and someone was shouting that I had a visitor. I called out, 'Fuck off. I don't want to see anybody. Go away.' But the hammering and banging went on and eventually I opened the door. The visitor was none other than the rock legend Eric Clapton. A real fucking legend. Not like me. And he'd come to see me? He said he'd heard I was here and that he'd been through a similar thing himself. I was so touched that he'd bothered to come and talk to me, and it helped a lot, just listening to his own experiences."

His denial, however, continued. After three weeks he was begging to get out.

> "As I began to feel a bit better, I took part in various activities. I organised five-a-side football games and quite enjoyed myself. I felt safe at the Priory. But at the same time, I still did not believe I was an alcoholic, so I did not accept what they said about me or the ways they were trying to help me.

> I should have stayed there longer. Everyone told me that, Bryan as well as all the experts, but I was fed up with it. I didn't think it was doing much for me. They didn't seem to really understand my problems. Or perhaps I wasn't giving them a proper chance."

Gazza went back again in 2002.

***

It was in November 1998 that Kate Moss checked into The Priory. It followed the collapse of her relationship with Johnny Depp and her drink and drug taking spiralling out of control. Her intention was to stay for two weeks but she stayed for five weeks. She later reflected that it was 'like boarding school', and she loved it.

Laura Collins, in her book *Kate Moss the Complete Picture* says "Tellingly, part of what she 'loved' was meeting 'normal' people. 'I did that whole walking in with dark glasses thing', she said, 'but after five minutes it felt ludicrous.' Not surprisingly, her stay at The Priory only increased her fascination. As Julie Burchill put it the following spring, Kate Moss was 'one of the most singular and shimmering icons this damp little island has ever produced'.

As Pene Dob relates later (see the chapter *A Spiritual Slant*), when Kate Moss joined her Priory yoga class she remembered thinking, *what a stunning girl, she should be a model*. It is difficult to imagine how Pene had missed all the hoo-ha about Kate in the media but not unusual within the disposition of Priory staff. They are not particularly interested in or bowled over by 'celebrity'. Pene took matters further - she avoided seeing patients' files, avoided knowledge of what anyone was 'in' for - let alone whether they were famous. She wanted no preconceived ideas in her classes.

***

Journalist Alan Franks wrote a feature in *The Times Magazine* in October '98 *The Last Chance Saloon,* about Galsworthy Lodge. He had been a patient there himself 11 years earlier, having 'ground to a halt with alcohol abuse'. Sitting in the programme, he was reminded what long, hard days they are on the unit. He sought out Chris Ball to ask her to explain the essence of what they were trying to achieve. Chris said:

> "The part that group therapy plays in this is to help people find within themselves a glimpse of someone who can relate and communicate with others without that terrible additive. There is no set subject matter, no set time for discussing a particular thing. So there always seems to be this unknown quantity about it, just as there is in life. That is the purpose of it, to draw people back in after the isolation of alcohol."

Dr David Craggs, the unit's Medical Director, added:

> "Of course there is still raging denial in some cases, but there is

less resistance than there used to be. As you go on studying this condition, the more you become aware of the emotional disconnection of the drinker, the fact that they are in another land."

Alan Franks concludes by recalling his own recovery and how the process is meant to be a partly spiritual affair. He says:

"I myself have remained on the 'darker' side of agnosticism. When other recovering addicts talk about the "Higher Power" which keeps them well, I listen like an envious boy. Still, the idea of some thing stronger than the individual should not be hard to accommodate for anyone who has been tyrannised by a substance or a liquid. The freedom from that tyranny is often described as a kind of heaven, and personally I would not have missed it for the earth."

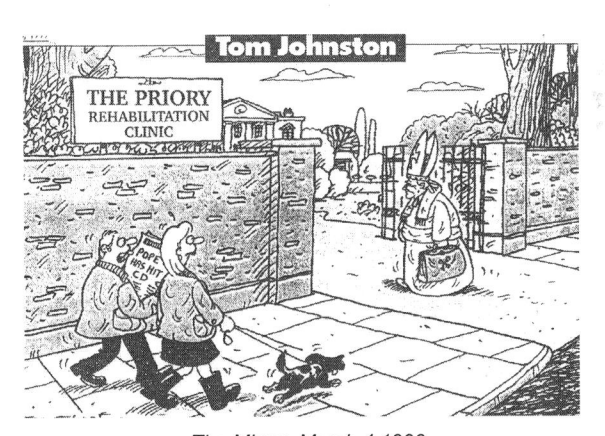

***

The Mirror, March 4 1999

When did I first realise that my son Rob was an alcoholic? I think it was a gradual process and perhaps my Priory antennae started twitching. I did know that my own consumption of alcohol went up when I was with him. We would share a bottle of wine with a meal, and he would precede this with a couple of beers, and more afterwards. And I was sure that he drank more when he wasn't with me. *Young people just drink a lot these days* was how I tried to comfort myself.

His letters described evenings spent with friends playing chess and going to the pub, the constant factors being booze and pot. I recalled the social worker's mention of his 'stormy and prolonged adolescence', and knew from what Rob had told me himself that things had not been easy.

Rob's relationship with alcohol started at the age of 12, when he would smuggle vodka into school. He left home when he was 15 and got into trouble with debts and bailiffs, fines and driving bans, fallings out at work, arguments with girlfriends. My head would spin with it all and he probably didn't tell me the half of it. When things were really bad, I wouldn't hear from him for weeks or months. I am convinced that working at The Priory helped me cope with what was happening to Rob, to us, because it was reflected in patients' stories, in the daily round of things. Although I had become something of a realist, I never stopped worrying. That's what Mums do.

Rob went to the Max Glatt Unit, a centre for drug and alcohol rehabilitation, in the mid-Nineties. Then in 2005, I was at work (in local government) when he phoned me. He had broken up with his girlfriend, he couldn't go on, and his slurred words were saying goodbye. I rushed up to my boss to say I had to go – my son might have taken an overdose.

Looking back, this must have surprised the poor lady on two levels. In orderly town halls you don't hear about overdoses too often. What's more, she hadn't known I had a son.

Mel, my soon-to-be-husband, drove us to Rob's flat, having first called for an ambulance to go there. Our journey took at least an hour and when we arrived Rob was absolutely furious with us. Two police cars and two ambulances had arrived at his flat and the police had "taken my ganj". His coffee table was strewn with vodka bottles, and a load of prescription drugs made out to other people. I didn't let myself think about where he got it all from. "Please let us take you to hospital", Mel pleaded, and to our amazement he agreed.

After waiting an interminable time in a side room at the hospital, a psychiatrist came to explain that they had to turn away several suicidal alcoholics a day. When he had finished speaking, Mel said "You've just spent 10 minutes telling us what you can't do. Now please tell us what you *can* do." The answer was nothing, and by this time Rob had sloped off home to drink.

When we returned from honeymoon in May 2006, Rob was in a desperate state. We took him to the TTP Counselling Centre in Luton, where he would undergo detox and rehabilitation. We fervently hoped it would save his life.

He settled into the programme and each time we visited during his rehab he seemed positively zealous about it all and looked 100% better.

12
I Don't Want To See You Again!
(in the nicest possible way)

Dianne Mackay, Admissions Manager
Priory Years: 1988 – ongoing

> Dianne runs the Admissions Department and her down-to-earth approach has calmed many an anxiety. She and I used to have a fine arrangement for the giving and receiving of goodies. For the most part, she gave and I received. The scheme only worked when her office was below mine, when I was able to rig up a basket and lower it on a long piece of rope to her office window. The basket would idly hang around until she took it in. Anticipation had me licking my lips, and sometimes I'd get biscuits or sweets. Other times I'd pull up that darned basket only to find a rude, inedible message inside.

"I had just been made redundant from a job near Oxford Street. I had always wanted to work in the medical world and there was an advert in the local newspaper. When I arrived for the interview, I couldn't believe the size and beauty of the building. I thought *there's no way someone like me can work somewhere like this*.

The interview was with Marianne Kelly from Admissions, and the Accounts Manager. I took to Marianne straight away but I didn't think it was going to happen. It must have been a Friday because when I was on my way home, she phoned and left a message with my Dad to say that they were keen and wanted me to start the following week! My Dad said, 'Oh you're going to like working with that Marianne, she's lovely.' And he was right. I wasn't so fond of the accounts side of things but dealing with the patients was very interesting. I didn't think anything of working in the private sector because I didn't know what it was like working for the NHS. My view was (and is) that if you can pay to get your health better then why not?

It was everything I expected in some respects. You had the doctors to look up to and it was like walking into a family. Everyone was so welcoming and kind. The nursing staff taught me about the Mental Health Act and about how to be with patients. Marianne did quite a few of the admissions with me at first but not long after I started she went on holiday and I had to do about three weeks on my own. I actually enjoyed the challenge.

Still, I was only 21 and there was a fear of the unknown. I was taught that when I checked in with the nurses before seeing a patient, they would alert me to anything I needed to know. But on one occasion they didn't tell me and I got a shock when I saw the patient, who was quite disfigured. I walked out of there thinking that I could never do that again. I don't know if the nurses forgot to tell me or maybe they didn't want to scare me.

Shortly after I started we had a young lady with a very strange condition, which I've never seen since – she could see bananas with spiders crawling on them. Another one was a patient who thought she was a dog. I suppose that's the most bizarre admission I've ever done in that she wanted to go to the ward on all fours. Actually, that was one of my quickest admissions. You do get used to it eventually but you never get blasé.

When you're on the front line like that, you don't know what the patient is going to be like. One minute they can be fine and then they can change. But those are rare cases and people are normally quite straightforward.

Admitting patients with alcohol or drug related problems can be difficult. The worst case was when someone vomited all over me. But mostly it's to do with the financial side of things. They might not remember, so you have to go back after a couple of days to go through things again.

Dr Shur always laughed at me because if someone well-known comes in, I usually don't have a clue who they are. I can only remember one occasion when somebody came in who was in a group that I liked when I was a teenager, and I made a complete fool of myself because I was so star struck. And his credit card was declined.

I can remember showing a patient around for Dr Shur, who was quite excited afterwards. He said 'Do you know who that was?' I hadn't a clue so he brought in an album cover to show me. In some ways it's a good thing I don't know who they are. And I get frustrated if people treat them differently; I think everybody should be treated the same.

A patient from 15 years back phoned recently as if we'd just spoken yesterday. He was in a very bad state. He was talking whilst drinking and then put the phone down on the floor and said he'd be back in a minute. I could hear him pouring himself another drink. We were on the phone for 45 minutes. He was scared he was going to die. We did get him in but unfortunately he had to be transferred.

Seeing the patients well enough to leave is why I still do the job. It's why I love being there. They are walking out of that door and they've got a smile back on their face. I sometimes joke with them, saying 'I don't want to see you again!' (in the nicest possible way, obviously)

The best/worst relationship I ever had with a patient was when I worked shifts one Christmas. A young anorexic girl would often come and sit in reception and have a chat. All the other girls were going home for Christmas or at least having some time out and she wasn't. She was such a sweet kid. It was one of the best things because I'd see her smile and she was happy by the time she left, when she was back to a healthy weight. The worst part was that I've never known what happened to her afterwards. They did a survey a couple of years ago of past patients and she was one who didn't respond. So that is the sad bit – never really knowing what happens.

I became the manager of the department about 15 years ago, and there was a time when I was running reception as well. You have to make sure that you look after the staff and that they have sufficient training and support.

One of the biggest things for me was when the four of us – Virginia [Pharmacist], Frances [Therapist], you Dorothy [P.A.], and I started our accountability group. The support we gave each other was probably the best thing that came out of the outward bound trip to Wales. We had regular lunches – often using Dr Kelly's office, which he didn't seem to mind – we even celebrated my 30th in Dr Kelly's office. We had some tough times at The Priory and the nice thing was that it wasn't just an accountability group for what was going on at work; it was about each of us as individuals. After you left Dotty, we still met up and encouraged each other about meeting blokes, marriage, birth, divorce…

It felt as though we were family then, and now the family is smaller. I'm so loyal and passionate about the Roehampton Priory and it was the people that made me feel that way.

My sense of humour I think does help on the basis that it can get tough and it can be sad and very stressful. There's no better way to sort that out than to have a giggle. I don't think I've ever laughed so much as when we formed the Fun Committee and arranged all those events. Our planning meetings were hilarious, trying to arrange what people would do, but the night we did *Blind Date*… well. To see Dr Shur, bless him, flapping about his flipping nails. It pops into my head at the weirdest moments: *Dr Shur, I did your makeup*! And the way people reacted that night – it was one of the funniest things ever.

There are times when I think I must move on – I've been here a very long time. But the minute you think *that's it, I can't do this anymore,* something comes along and you feel like you're doing something to help somebody. There was a difficult patient last week and everyone said someone's going to have to sit down and talk to this woman. I said I'll do it and at the end the patient said, 'I like you. You know what you're talking about.' That's the reason I'm there – it's the patients, the consultants and the colleagues."

13
Sanctuary

This chapter includes patients' own stories, and excerpts from autobiographies and biographies. The description 'sanctuary' has been used by many patients over the years about The Priory.

Every staff member will tell you that the most wonderful thing about working at The Priory is the patients. You know that you are in the company of original, creative minds; minds so enviable yet they can be so fragile.

Thinking of the early days (at least as far as this record is concerned), Professor Michael Gelder, who chaired a seminar in June '99, revealed that he had worked at The Priory himself, in 1958. His first impression was of pastoral parkland, cows, and a milkmaid. He described the inside of the building as being in a state of 'shabby gentility'. The hospital was going through a difficult period, with a medical superintendent who had been unwell for several years, but Dr John Flood had just become the new medical director.

One extremely well-dressed patient the young Dr Gelder met on his first day had a lady's maid occupying the room next door; she too had been admitted three years previously. And this was a time, he recalled, when some patients would stay at The Priory for a few weeks, move on for a leucotomy operation at nearby Atkinson Morley's Hospital, then come back again. He met one of these patients, a Middle Eastern gentleman, during his first ward round. In fact he all but fell over the man's servant, who was lying on a mat at the foot of his master's bed, armed with a large dagger.

When Community Psychiatric Centers bought The Priory in September 1980, there were about 20 acute and 50 psychogeriatric patients (long stay). By the time I joined the staff in 1982, the remaining long stay patients were predominantly female and not a little quirky. Some didn't leave their rooms much (if at all) and a select few had their own private nurses.

Two patients had specific tasks in the daily running of the hospital. I'm not sure how long they had held down these responsibilities (let alone how they came about) but they took their roles very seriously indeed.

Mrs C ran the hospital shop. This was a part-time affair housed in a sort of cupboard on one of the wards. Mrs C liked to do things properly and doing things properly took time. She would count out change with all the solemnity of a religious rite, while a patient queue formed in front of her. As a staff member, your own needs might be a quick Kit-Kat to elevate your energy but frustration elevated your blood pressure instead. What was worse was if Mrs C spotted you in the queue: "Make way!" she commanded the waiting patients. "Staff member! Busier than you!" Mortified, you'd slink away, vowing never to give in to a chocolate craving again.

Then there was Mrs G, who organised the Sunday Services in the Chapel. In preparation, she would clean the silver and make sure the chairs were positioned perfectly. Every August she would appear in the Secretariat with a list of next year's services painstakingly prepared. This must now be typed and when to her liking, a box of fruit jellies would be placed on one of our desks.

One patient would slap my desk in times of need. Dr Kelly was not her doctor but this didn't matter a hoot. 'I don't want to be buried at sea', she might begin, followed by some heavy breathing and a meaningful pause, 'I can't swim.' I would hasten to reassure her that no one could possibly have it in mind to bury her at sea, but she was ready for that: 'I don't want a communist's death either.' Another day it would be, 'Will you tell Dr Kelly I don't want euthanasia in five years.' Sometimes I would try a pro-active approach: 'How can I help you today?' only to be told 'You can't. This is a Jewish problem.' Thus let off the hook, I would return to my work and she would continue on her worried way.

John Hughes remembers another long stay patient, a Major 'H':

> "He was quite a personality who lived to be about 100 at The Priory. He had a First World War canvas bag, a sort of rucksack that he always carried. It was dirty and in shreds. He was in the trenches in the First World War, had battlefield fatigue and a breakdown. The story was that he murdered his batman. He was immediately filed away as a psychiatric case in a state hospital.
>
> A firm of solicitors continued to collect the Major's army salary - later a disability pension - which accumulated interest in a trustee account for fifty years. When his initial solicitor died or retired, someone younger in the firm took over the Major's case. They realised that this chap had several hundred thousand pounds accumulated and had never spent anything while in state hospitals. So they moved Major 'H' from one of the state psychiatric hospitals in Surrey – they didn't have the military ones any more by then – and decided that he should finish his days in a nice place like The Priory."

Not everyone is keen to spend time at The Priory and a little persuasion is required. Joyce Herrmann, the maintenance chief's wife, told me about when she was working in Reception - it would have been in the Fifties or Sixties.

> "I had a message that a very famous star was arriving from Heathrow for admission. She had smuggled a kitten into the country and wouldn't be parted from it. The only way she could stay in England was if she agreed to become a patient at The Priory. But when she arrived here she created the most awful furore. She said she was not going to stay in this ghastly place and that she wasn't mad darlink! I was getting very anxious by this time and there was only one doctor she would allow near her. He said to me, "Don't worry. I lay odds I will have her at my feet in 15 minutes." He won his bet: a loud thump pronounced her sedated."

Sanctuary

It was during the Sixties that the number of singers, musicians and film stars finding their way to The Priory door escalated. Paul Robeson, the American singer and actor, was admitted under the Mental Health Act in September 1961, following a suicide attempt. Robeson and his wife Ellie were greeted at the door by Dr Flood. "HE is our man," Ellie wrote to a friend. "He is Paul's choice and he and Dr Ackner are the ONLY ones he talks to."

As Martin Bauml Duberman relates in the biography *Paul Robeson*, he was suffering from what Priory Consultant Brian Ackner referred to as 'one of those somewhat rare chronic depressions which fail to respond to any therapy or continue to relapse but which in the long run have a good prognosis.' Dr Flood supported this view, although he referred to it as 'endogenous depression in a manic depressive personality'. They put their patient on a drug and ECT regime that initially brought him out of a 'down' cycle, encouraging the doctors to continue the regime.

Mr Robeson was an inpatient for many months. Hordes of reporters took to waiting at both Priory entrances; some were chased from the grounds, others even infiltrated the wards. By August 1963, the press harassment was so bad that it was decided that Robeson should be transferred to a clinic in Berlin. Inevitably, his departure had to be a cloak and dagger affair, with his wife Ellie having to disguise herself to leave their flat in Connaught Square, while Mr Robeson was secreted out of The Priory on the floor of a car.

Cleaner and tea lady Doris Day, a huge admirer of Mr Robeson, remembers his stay very well.

> "When Mr Robeson was a patient, I was desperate to have a good look at him, so I spoke to the cleaner who did his room and pleaded with her to let me go in instead. So she gave me her duster and I dusted around a bit then went over to his bed. There was a little bedside table and I was trying to dust between all the stuff on there, while having a look at him. I knocked over a bottle of whisky! Oh, it was terrible. He had hidden it there and must have drunk about half, and the rest spilled all over the floor. He was *furious*."

***

In 1965, the author and artist Mervyn Peake, who had written *Titus Groan* and *Gormenghast*, was admitted after a degenerative neurological disease (a form of Parkinson's Disease) had left him unable to write or paint. The hospital, by now in a state of visible neglect, must have presented a formidable sight to the new arrival. His biographer, John Watney in *Mervyn Peake*, compared The Priory to a "cut-price Victorian version of Gormenghast", referring to its "...tall, massive, grey structure, with a few windows punched indiscriminately in it and a medieval-style door." But he had previously been at Banstead Hospital and his wife Maeve swore she would never let him go to a place like that again.

The Priory charged around £118 a month, which the family could ill-afford, "Yet this," wrote Watney, "was the only place for Mervyn. Here he was cared for and looked after. Here was comfort and civilisation."

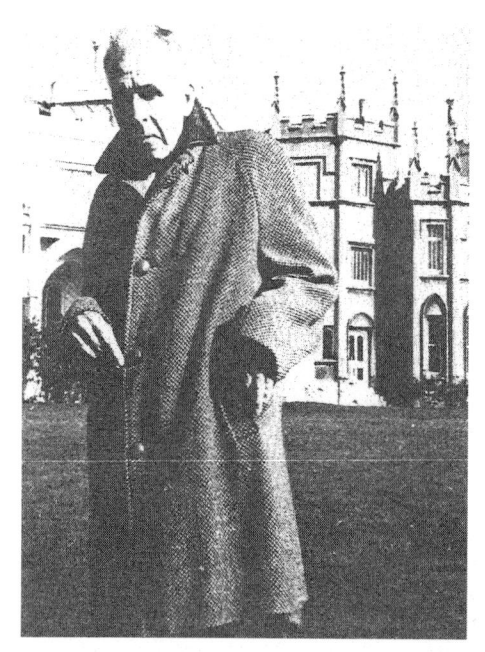

Photo taken by Fabian Peake in the grounds of The Priory

Later in the Sixties, and desperate for money, the governors of The Priory decided that a portion of the grounds must be sold to a development company, meaning that the wing where Mr Peake had his room would be demolished. Some of the patients were men who had been wounded in the Great War of 1914-18; others were 'pop' stars who had found the going too hard.

It was in March 1968 that Mr Peake was taken to his brother-in-law's nursing home, where he died on 16 November that year.

***

When he was at the height of his success, John Ogdon, a world famous British pianist, had a series of breakdowns. In 1973, having submitted to (and escaped from) the horrors of a hospital resembling 'Bedlam', John Ogdon was admitted to The Priory which, by contrast, was luxurious and cosy.

His wife Brenda Lucas, in the book she wrote with Michael Kerr – *Virtuoso: The Story of John Ogdon* - tells how she felt compelled to ask the doctor who would be looking after her husband – 'Doctor, he isn't insane, is he?' 'Temporarily insane', he said gently. For her 'temporarily' was the word that mattered. Told the next day that there could be no hope for John without a course of electric shock treatment (for which she would have to give permission), she asked for time to decide. Finding the burden too much to handle alone, she went home to phone some of their closest friends. He was, after all, not only her husband but an outstanding musician and public figure. After two days of doubt and delay, she gave her reluctant permission. As she later reasoned: "An artist, however outstanding, is also a man – and a million times better a sane healthy man than a great talent locked in a cell!" Suicide attempts and further breakdowns brought John Ogdon back to The Priory again and again, with a paranoid schizo-affective psychosis.

I understand that he used to play the grand piano in the chapel.

***

It was the mid-Eighties when Spike Milligan told his agent and manager Norma Farnes, 'I need to go to my Alma Mater.' In her book *Spike An Intimate Memoir*, Ms Farnes continues:

> "He said he was in a constant state of panic, could not sleep and was walking round the house at two and three in the morning. By the end of the week he was in his alma mater, the Priory at Roehampton. It was a very quiet Milligan who came out of the Priory after a period of deep narcosis, the chemically induced sleep he occasionally resorted to. The entry in my diary for this time reads, 'Spike is so quiet. It's not normal. "Yes" to everything.' A manic depressive, Spike Milligan's crazy humour was born of his highs but paid for by his lows."

***

A Consultant Physician was admitted to The Roehampton Priory in 1986 and gives this account of his stay:

"I had been working as a doctor in the Middle East for four years, which my wife and I viewed as a temporary posting prior to returning to the UK with our three small children. Before taking this Middle East posting I had been offered a dream UK job for which I had planned in detail to take up on return to the UK. This was suddenly withdrawn, precipitating a mental and emotional crisis with my deepest hopes dashed. It provoked great puzzlement in the local oil company context in the Gulf. Apparently, I exhibited great self-control which led to multiple possible diagnoses during hospitalisation in Auckland, New Zealand and in London.

To this day, I remember the quiet yet authoritative confidence emanating from Desmond Kelly with what appeared to me even in my distressed state to be sensible strategies. This reassurance greatly strengthened my wife and my parents.

The surroundings were posh but it was the care that made me better. There was no history of bipolar disorder for me or my family. There was considerable talking through my inner turmoil and it seemed to be aimed at helping me to understand myself rather than some academic exercise for the professionals. I was grateful for people with technical expertise but it was that combination with kindness that got me on the road to recovery.

I guess that even in my fragility I wanted a clear outcome fast. It was not only the pills that slowed me down but the calm sanctuary of sympathetic staff. A safe place in which to work these things through is vital.

The art of knowing when someone is ready on their journey to re-enter the rough and tumble of real life is not easily addressed in the textbooks. The Priory and Dr Kelly in particular, demonstrated that clinical skill in persuading me to stay when I was reluctant and then giving me and the family confidence to re-enter normal life at the appropriate moment.

I was eighteen months out of work. I was given a role by a Chief Medical Officer in a major national unit. She was passionate about minimising the stigma of mental illness in the workplace and I think her confidence in me was not misplaced since a speciality career has flourished over the last twenty years.

I have subsequently received excellent care in the NHS and have been a good boy taking my Lithium. I still contribute some innovative ideas but in a more measured way!

I remain ever grateful that there was expertise and kindness at The Priory when I needed it in my most florid state."

***

As name after name checked in, the hospital came to be seen by the media as a significant qualification on a celebrity CV, despite the fact that only the genuinely ill referred by a doctor would be admitted. When the *Daily Express* compiled a Londoners A-Z of snobbery in 1987, 'P' was for The Priory, 'the Blenheim Palace of mental hospitals', 'a last social oasis where the rich and socially ambitious can't always gain admission.'

Some people have absolutely no intention of gaining admission. A psychiatrist remembers approaching his car, ready to leave one day when a man appeared and said 'Are you going towards Putney? Could I have a lift?' The doctor said 'Of course'. Afterwards he remembers having spotted Dr Kelly standing in the car park, staring after them and as he reached the Upper Richmond Road, he began to sense that something was particularly wrong. It dawned on him that this gentleman was perhaps not a bona fide passenger. At his attempt to make a quick u-turn back to the hospital, the man said 'Thanks very much, I'll get out here' and leapt out of the car. The Consultant later learned that Desmond Kelly had just spent two hours trying to admit the man.

***

Nicola

Another lady who had no intention of staying was the beautiful actress Nicola Pagett, perhaps best known for her role in the original television series *Upstairs Downstairs.* She gives a remarkable account of manic depressive illness (or bipolar disease) in her 1997 book *Diamonds Behind My Eyes.* She becomes obsessed with the Prime Minister's press secretary Alastair Campbell ('The Stranger' in her book) and her subsequent experiences as an inpatient at The Priory are described painfully, honestly, and at times hilariously. Desmond Kelly (who is 'Dr Darling', while The Priory is 'the Sanctuary') wrote the Afterword, explaining that manic depressive illness...

> "...has two dramatic faces, like the bright and dark sides of the moon. In the manic phase, the brain is racing until it spins out of control. Thoughts come cascading out, with irresistible pressure, until reason is drowned in the torrent of swirling ideas. The mind loses its balance and generates garbage data. The senses are heightened, there is rising optimism, over-confidence, and often an exaggerated mood of romance that is compelling and all-consuming. Because the mental linkages are so fast, other people's thinking seems pedestrian, and the consequent impatience and irritability is a hallmark of the condition.
>
> Any suggestion that this active, super-charged state could be an illness is naturally dismissed out of hand. As Sigmund Freud put it so well, 'Illusions commend themselves to us because they save us pain and allow us to enjoy pleasure instead. We must therefore accept it without complaint when they sometimes collide with a bit of reality against which they are dashed to pieces.' The pleasure is intense and the illusion is that it can go on forever; therefore when reality intrudes there is an explosion of complaint..."

As Nicola Pagett began to get better, she realised that...

> "It wasn't a spooky place, the Sanctuary, people were just people. They weren't particularly mad, they were just broken.
>
> I hate going to 'improve thyself' gatherings, but I thought I'd better go to a few. If I really behave, I thought, they might let me out. I started having long, boring conversations with rather old ladies suffering from depression – so they could see how charitable I was. In fact, whenever there were doctors or nurses about, I made a point of being absolutely adorable to everybody. I went to a flower-arranging class run by the cheeriest of cheerful souls it has ever been my misfortune to meet. She was so enchanting I wanted to smash her face in. When your life's in bits on the floor the last thing you need is to be grinned at all the time.
>
> My God, I thought, I'm normal again. Even though I do not know anything about arranging fucking flowers – I'll bloody well do it.

The cheery lady was smiling away and chattering. I kept sticking all these flowers into the wire. It didn't look very good. In fact it looked terrible. But the whole thing was getting gratifyingly bigger. There were yawning gaps, though; my creation seemed to have too many holes. We'd all been allocated a certain amount of flowers, and I don't know what came over me, but I nicked my neighbour's Sweet Williams. She was having a vague sort of day and I knew she wouldn't notice. So as a result my flower erection looked absolutely brilliant and it was placed in reception. Every time I walked past it, I got a huge thrill."

***

Michael

"I had a nervous breakdown in 1979. We lived in Mayfair then, and an ambulance took me to Bowden House because The Priory was full.

Later, when I first went to The Priory, I had actually wanted to go to Switzerland. We had been skiing and met some people who knew Professor Kielholz and said, 'Go and see him; he's excellent.' I knew he was looking after royalty at the time and thought *if he's good enough for them*. But Professor Kielholz advised that it would be much easier for me to go and see Desmond Kelly at The Priory, than travel backwards and forwards to Switzerland. That made sense and I've been at The Priory quite a few times now.

I couldn't come to terms with what was wrong with me. I couldn't understand it. Depression? I'd never been depressed in my life.

I'd always had excellent jobs. When my partner and I met, I was the manager of a large group of hair salons in London and Rome. He was in banking and worked for Rothschilds. Then we thought *this is ridiculous, we may as well have a business of our own,* and that's how we started the first hair salon in Belgravia. He did the bookwork and I sorted out the logistics, the staff, and did the hair. That was in 1978, and we opened other salons in hotels. But then I got this depression thing and couldn't cope with the staffing and just wouldn't go into work sometimes.

So in about 1983 we went to look at The Priory. When Desmond Kelly showed us around, it stood out as a magnificent building; like a castle. We were very impressed.

I was diagnosed as manic depressive. In those days it wasn't called bipolar, it was manic depression. Then it was bipolar or unipolar. Unipolar is when you're down all the time. Bipolar is when you swing up and down.

Sister Renée, on Garden Wing, was excellent. She wasn't a hard woman but was very firm and knew exactly what she was doing. I liked her very much and we got on like a house on fire. She would help me unpack and say, 'Oh, he's got Gucci belts and Gucci shoes!'

I liked a particular room and whenever I came back and they didn't have that room, Renée would fix it. She'd say 'Michael, I know you're not going to be happy.' The last time I went there I was very unhappy. The room they gave me was facing the nurses' station and I couldn't cope with that. Also, the bedspread and curtains didn't match and the curtains didn't close. I opened the wardrobe door and it fell off its hinges. So that was all changed within 24 hours.

I'm very sensitive you see. This has always been my problem, even as a child at boarding school. I've always been very particular and everything has to be just so. And this is a killer because it can't always be like that in life. I don't know what it is. Being an only child and having been brought up in a Jewish family and being given everything by my grandparents and my father. And with my mother being so ill… Later on in life, as a result, I always wanted the same thing. Fortunately, it happened. We're not rich but we're comfortable. People say you've got this and that, and I say 'What do material things mean? It's how you feel inside.'

I couldn't cope with the fact that my mother wasn't walking. She was ill in bed for 10 years. I'd say, 'Get in your wheelchair Mum and I'll take you to Grandma's,' but she wouldn't let anyone see her in her wheelchair. She just stayed in bed. She had the worst type of multiple sclerosis and died at the age of 46.

I didn't take part in the activities available at The Priory, I didn't feel like it. I used to go to Richmond Park and walk quite a lot, when I was allowed to. I didn't mix much in the therapy classes but I used to go to the yoga, which was relaxing and soothing and put you at peace with yourself.

I found the therapy sessions very good, until I had a problem. There were about 20 people in the class and they were asking various questions, all around the room. There was a biggish woman there, not very attractive, but that's beside the point. She wanted me to be friendly with her but I didn't want to be. I didn't want anything to do with her, she drove me mad. She was saying how her husband left her and I know I shouldn't have said it, but I said 'Well look at you. Do you wonder why he's left you?' She said, 'What's wrong with me?' And I said, 'Find a mirror.'

She went bananas, screamed and cried. They got hold of Desmond Kelly and he said 'What have you done? I was supposed to come out that day and I was so nervous that he was going to keep me in. I said 'Please don't say I've got to stay longer.' He said 'I'm not, but I'll have to put you on different medication. You were very strong with this woman; she's in a terrible state. You've put her right back.'

I had a problem with another woman too. She was making terrible noises in the dining room. I won't tell you what I said but we took our plates and moved tables. Her husband was there and said he was going to kill me. So I said, 'Do it, please!' One of the doctors said he thought it would be best if I apologised to her, that she was erratic, she'd come for me in the night. That made me bloody nervous because you can't lock the doors! I met her a couple of times going into the dining room and she was spitting at me, so a day or so later I went to her room, knocked on the door, and said I'd come to apologise. It was all my fault and I didn't mean it. She was all right then.

I remember an occasion when I had been allowed out for the evening and was dropped back at The Priory around midnight. I rang the bell for 15 minutes but nobody came, even though I had told them I was going to be late. So I decided to knock on one of the patient's windows. This guy was in a deep sleep and thought somebody had come to take him away (it's true that I was trying to get in the window at one stage). He shouted 'Take me! Take me!' I don't know what he'd been dreaming about but he complained that I ruined it. All these heads were coming out of windows and eventually a depressed patient let me in. It must have been about 1am by then. The patients were all shaking on the ground floor; they came out of their rooms and the nurse offered them hot drinks. I just casually went to my room and to bed. I was exhausted!

If I feel well, the world is my oyster, I can do anything. But when you're really ill, being at The Priory makes you feel cushioned. Everything is done for you and you feel secure and safe. I know it's no good to be hospitalised but you definitely feel better in surroundings like that, and you can relate to the other people.

But afterwards, when I used to see Desmond as an outpatient, we sometimes ended up laughing for half an hour. Because what is there to talk about?

You're either low or you're not low."

***

In July 1987, a 26 year old Canadian student came over to be reviewed for leucotomy. I don't think DK had ever encountered anyone quite as sick in terms of his obsessional cleanliness. He had obsessive-compulsive disorder (OCD) and had been housebound for years, his main human contact being his parents. Nothing could be touched without plastic gloves, his showers took hours and all his belongings had to be placed methodically. He believed that if he touched something dirty the very essence of that thing would become part of him, would kill him. Every treatment had been tried; he was suicidal and his parents, both scientists, were in despair. His Mum brought him to Desmond Kelly for help.

A lot of preparation went into the build-up for his interview with the Mental Health Act Commissioners. This was an essential step along the way to a leucotomy. They agreed that he should have surgery and he was taken to Atkinson Morley's Hospital in Wimbledon for the operation. It took ages to get him into the taxi for the short journey and when he arrived at AMH he couldn't get through the front entrance, where there was litter. I had a panic call from his Mum and sent a

Registrar over to help. Once over the hurdle of the entrance, he wouldn't get onto a bed until they had placed 26 sheets upon it.

The night before the operation he announced he couldn't go through with it; he returned to The Priory, to the airport and to the States. To say we were all terribly disappointed would be an understatement. DK was very distracted, convinced the young man would go back to the States and kill himself.

The following October we had a phone call: he wanted to try again. This time we sent him an operation consent form to sign before travelling. And this time he even managed a touch of humour on the eve of the op. Gazing at DK while he wrote his customarily impenetrable 'to do' lists, overlaid with unfathomable aide-memoires, the patient ventured, 'Don't you think you're being a bit obsessional?'

The operation went very well and he returned to The Priory in the November. Now the real work began. We non-medical staff didn't see much of him for a while and then he began to show up in the dining room and wandered around talking to people. He was undergoing intensive behaviour therapy and faced hefty challenges. The outside world was threatening, hostile and infinitely filthy but at least he was open to the idea of *trying* now. He even made an appearance at the Christmas party, which must have been a huge ordeal. I had watched him sometimes. When spotting a particularly unsavoury looking person ahead, on a ward or corridor, he would about-heel and rush off in the opposite direction until the danger had gone. And who could blame him?

He began to appear in my office, sit down and wait for something to happen. I had two options; either I could ignore him or I could chat, try to give him confidence, draw him out. He didn't have much practical experience of life; he had done his living through reading books. So we talked about books. His father had introduced him to the writing of Iris Murdoch. I'm a fan of hers too. I took the risk of offering to lend him a couple of books, knowing this would be difficult for him (reading a used book) but he accepted with a frown. 'Give it a go', I said, 'even if turning each page is hell.'

One evening when leaving work I saw him picking his way along the drive. It was dark and he was peering at the ground making sure not to tread on anything revolting, every fibre tensed. It was one of the most moving sights I've ever seen.

The first time I saw a slow smile break through a frown on his anxious face, I knew I had witnessed the sort of Priory miracle we all work there for. Doctors and staff alike became very fond of this patient. We all went the extra mile for him and he repaid us by the sheer effort he put into his recovery. I felt a particular empathy towards him I think because of my mother's OCD; he was also an extremely nice man.

When he returned to Canada he would send letters and poetry, and the following

Christmas I thought he might appreciate an audio tape of news and encouragement from all his friends back at The Priory. It was fantastic to see patients, nurses, therapists, doctors and other staff literally queuing to talk to him on tape, with others travelling miles to say their piece. It became a sort of celebration; they were all so pleased about his recovery, in which they had taken part. He had captured the imagination and affection of us all.

A section of his poem, The Souls' Diaspora – a wondrous odyssey through his family history - described the start of his illness at the age of twelve.

> ...and then the sickness
> came slouching forward.
> Anxiety. Obsession. A plague
> of blue notions. Mysterious detonations
> in the brain. A fortress dismayed by
> treason, thought assaulting reason, arrows
> shot from the inside, mental mud slides
> shaking the foundation of my learning...

He would never know easy contentment or be careless of the threats that surrounded him yet he retained a sense of humour, an abiding love of reading, a huge talent for writing and, post operation, a capacity to attempt the unthinkable. His courage was remarkable.

***

Dr Michael Trimble, the expert on Gilles de la Tourette Syndrome (based at the National Hospital for Nervous Diseases in Queen Square) asked Dr Kelly to see a couple of patients before and after limbic leucotomy. Both of these patients were exceptional in that they did not have the more usual symptoms of Tourette's, such as involuntary tics or bouts of foul language. One of them had a compulsion to touch the back of his eyeball with his finger. He would have been blind or dead in a year but after the operation he did very well.

The other man, who could not control his destructive urges (for example to smash glass or tear his clothes and blankets into ribbons) had a documentary made about him – *Cutting Edge: Against My Nature*, aired in April 1990 on Channel 4. They filmed his interviews with Dr Kelly, who said that people often asked him why operations such as leucotomy were still carried out. He explained that there are demonstrable structural changes in the brain with the Gilles de la Tourette Syndrome: it is an organic condition.

Mr Henry Marsh, the leading Neurosurgeon who would carry out the operation, described it like this:

> "The operation is called a Stereotactic Limbic Interruption (or 'Leucotomy', which I tend not to use because it has emotional overtones). It involves making a series of very small lesions (which means a destructive hole) in a very specific part of the brain called the limbic system. The limbic system is the part of the brain

that deals with emotion and arousal and the purpose of the operation is to damage the limbic system in two very small areas, thereby changing the patient's emotional balance and the level at which they become aroused and anxious."

Following his recovery from surgery and intensive behaviour therapy, the patient came back to see Dr Kelly for review. Again it was filmed and this time he brought along his long-suffering girlfriend. They seemed very sweet together as they sat whispering in the waiting room but as the programme revealed, their relationship was anything but straightforward. The last shot was of the couple walking across The Priory lawn, talking about a future together in a little place by the seaside. Sadly, the patient died of an unrelated heart attack 18 months post-operation.

Marianne

"I was there for 8 weeks. We have a home in Spain and that's where I became ill. I knew I had to get back to England because I didn't think I could cope with all that in Spanish. And because of the depression a lot of physical things were going wrong. My whole system was shutting down and I was desperate. So my husband, bless his cotton socks, got me on a plane. I couldn't look up or open my mouth anymore. Friends told us about Dr John Cobb and we went to see him at his rooms. He said 'The Priory' and we said 'But when?' Two hours later I was there.

When I saw the little room they were going to put me in, without an en-suite bathroom I thought *I can't stay*. I later understood that it was an observation room. My husband said 'That was the hardest thing to do, to walk away and leave you there.' I didn't get out of that room for four days, apart from to open my door and scoot along to the loo, then scoot back to my room with blankets over me. I just didn't want to see anyone. The number of times I begged Tom to take me home.

But I couldn't even get out of the gate, never mind make a dash for it. I found the place very confusing at first. You're already befuddled and there are all those corridors. It took me weeks to find my way to the front and get out in the garden. I was encouraged to go to the restaurant and I finally found it one day. I stood at the door and saw all these people getting on with it and went straight back to my room.

When I did manage to slink in, I sat at a little table at the back. A lady came over and said 'You look a bit lost. If you want somebody to listen, all you do is this...' and she climbed on a table and said 'We're here!' When she climbed down, she said 'I'm not allowed to associate with you because I'm in the Galsworthy programme. But come on, let's go and get you something to eat.' She was brilliant! Many a lunch I shared with her and we became pals. Sometimes she was with the whole gang from what I assume was Galsworthy. It wasn't until weeks later that someone said 'Don't you recognise her?' I don't know any famous faces; I'm useless with that sort of thing.

I felt a great need to have a pal at The Priory. A young girl was brought in around the same time as me and I felt so sorry for her because she was the same age as my children. We looked for one another on Upper Court, where there's that communal room. But it just shows you how vulnerable you are because in the room next to her came a lady more her age, and they struck a chord together. I felt very left out – I was quite tearful about it! Then a lady arrived in the room opposite me and she was my age, on my wavelength, and we have kept up.

I didn't like the group sessions where you all sit around and have to say something about yourself. I used to think *I don't mind talking to John Cobb but why should I confide in these people?* But I think they were good and I had total trust in the staff there: total.

I'm an organising sort of person and quite a logical thinker and I loved all the skill tests outside. For example, 12 people stand on a long plank and you have to sort yourselves out according to height, without touching the ground. It's very good as you have to have physical contact. You always find one or two leaders. Some people just stand there and wait to be told what to do and of course I'm so bossy. I said 'How am I going to get past you? Your tummy sticks out so I'd rather go round the back of you. Do you mind?!'

I liked the evening sessions that were just in your area because you got to know the other people there. One of the senior staff would come in and you would talk about what sort of a day you'd had, because we wouldn't all have been doing the same thing. You lose your inhibitions and chat openly. Someone would say 'I've had a shit day and all I could do was cry.' You'd think *wow, I'm not doing too badly then.*

I couldn't leave the grounds for a long time. Dr Cobb said 'Just go to the gate, look up the road towards the Park and you'll see a lamppost. Try and walk to that lamppost.' I did that with my husband a few times and that wasn't too bad. Then I did it on my own and got back feeling very wobbly. But I'd done it. Then one day when I knew roughly what time my husband would arrive at Barnes Station, I thought I'm going to surprise him, I'm jolly well going to get across that road. I stood there and he came off the train and his face was just…

Looking back, I think how ridiculous that it was difficult but it was! And even when you've left it goes on – it's little steps. I'm so lucky that it did all come back, *and* a lot of things better than before. I had a fear of heights. I've lost it! I can go to the top of the escalator in the underground and zoom all the way down, I can run down.

For the first four weeks, I couldn't let my children come near me. I don't know whether it was because I felt ashamed – I can't put my finger on it. When I eventually asked for them to pop in… it still brings tears to my eyes to think about it.

I thought I was going to die. I wanted to die. But I got through it. That's why I still see John Cobb, about once every nine months, because a) I really like him and b) because he's there.

My husband was away an awful lot before he retired, probably 60% of our married life he was abroad. So you just get on with it and because we'd always been like that I didn't know any different. When the boys were really young he came back from South Africa to Yorkshire and one month later he left for three years. He would come home every three months for three weeks and we would fight for a day because he thought I couldn't even unscrew a light bulb!

When we lived in Kent, I became Chairman of Governors of a big junior school and I would get up and talk to all these parents. People said 'oh, you're so confident', but inside I was like a jelly. I don't think I could do anything like that now but I hardly ever become like a jelly inside anymore so I'm on a much more even keel.

At one stage we had three homes – London, Guernsey and Spain. And then we sold London, sold Guernsey, bought another place in Spain, sold the apartment we had in Spain and it was three moves, organising all that, plus I had to cope with Spanish. And my husband – technical things he's wonderful – but not languages. And that's really what got me into The Priory. It was all on my shoulders and having three house moves in a year and having builders in for three months and trying to cope with them in a different language. So I'm not making that mistake again. We will do one thing at a time.

In the beginning, you can't wait to get away and then when they say you can leave, you're terrified. We came back to the flat and stayed here another three months before I felt ready to leave living near Dr Cobb! Then we went back to Spain.

Dr Cobb always says that clinical depression is just that you don't produce certain chemicals and that's why you have to take these pills. I quite like that. So I still take my medication. Dr Cobb says it's a very low dosage – 'You'll have to take it for the rest of your life and don't worry about it.'

It was good for me, The Priory, and I will always be grateful. They got me on the right path and they knew how to motivate me. But I tell you, my biggest fear is to go back to The Priory. I will do everything in my power not to go down that road."

***

When journalist John Crace was admitted to The Priory, he was convinced that he was dying from BSE [bovine spongiform encephalopathy, better known as mad-cow disease]. However, his newly found psychiatrist at The Priory said that in fact he was clinically depressed, and definitely did not have BSE.

Crace describes in his book *The Second Half: thoughts from a male mid-life crisis* that once he had settled in, he began to meet some of the other inmates on his wing, deciding that…

> "…by and large, a nicer group of nutters you couldn't hope to meet. OK, some of the more severe schizophrenics were a little tricky to hold down a conversation with, and the depressives who turned their chairs to face the wall weren't great company either, but there were plenty of others to hang out with. The manic depressives were usually the most fun. They had invariably been dragged kicking and screaming into the hospital after a manic binge, during which they had generally spent thousands of pounds they didn't have, and would pace up and down the corridors talking to anyone prepared to listen."

When the medication kicked in he realised he no longer had BSE, yet he was extremely reluctant to leave.

> "No one raised their voice, and everyone was enthusiastic, congratulatory and kind. Completely outside the realms of my normal experience. Mental hospital is the closest I have ever got to civilization."

***

Author, columnist and agony aunt, Virginia Ironside stayed at The Priory through two bouts of depression, and described her recurrent depression as a feeling of total isolation.

> "All those poor fools, running out being enthusiastic about going to birthday parties and going to the theatre, are living in a dream world. The truth is life is hell… I feel as if there is an enormous piece of glass between me and the rest of the world: sometimes it is double glazing."

Ironside also said that she…

> "…couldn't think of a better place to be when one feels that life isn't worth living any more.", noting that she didn't see anyone glamorous at The Priory and wanted to dispel the myth that it was a place where star guests went for a bit of pampering. "This is a complete fiction. The truth is that everyone there is suffering. But if you have to suffer, I'd prefer to suffer at The Priory than anywhere else."

Ruby

"Dr Mark Collins saved my life by saying I had clinical depression. I had no idea up until that point; we thought I had glandular fever or something, we couldn't figure out what it was. Then Mark declared it clinical depression and I wept with joy.

So as soon as my daughter was born, Mark knew to get me into The Priory. I was so befuddled that I ended up at a betting shop in Richmond, because that's where I assumed The Priory was. I was carrying pyjamas and a toothbrush. Luckily, the people at the betting shop drove me to the right place. Those nurses were the mother I never had. It was childhood, and they took me into a warm room and it was sort of like returning to the womb. It was love.

But I rambled on about tennis lessons and needing to go to the gym to do my sit ups and could I use the phone and really someone crazier than me should be using this room. The nurse was all warm and lovely and giving me a cup of tea and then the doctor shoots me up with a syringe. So I was out for the next two days or so and then when I woke up, gradually, I was with my people."

Ruby talks about what happened next in her book *How do you want me?*

> "Gradually, a curiosity long buried perks up its head and you wonder, who else is here? So reluctantly you foray like a frightened dog into the cafeteria with the feelings you had when you were eight, that no one will want to sit with you. But you, like a brave little soldier, go in just like your first day at nursery school, and one kind soul says can they sit next to you? And you're shy and grateful, but can't find the old shtick you used to spin the magic with. The person looks the way you feel and you tell them that you don't know what to eat, or say, or look like and they say, 'Me too.' And there it is: finally you are with your tribe."

Back in our conversation, she continues:

"At first I wouldn't leave my room at all – they bring the food to you – but I adored the nurse: it was total bonding. Whichever nurse I had, I loved her. Of course, it was a mother substitute and that was why I was in The Priory in the first place. Then I started mingling with people and they were always the most glorious people I have ever met because of course they had my illness.

And no one can be more amusing about their own illness than a depressive. Don't forget that it usually hits the brightest and that's the irony, because we're all in there thinking we're idiots. And it's not any particular class – that's why I always hate it when people say you have to be privileged to have depression.

We would all go outside and have to be a farm animal. We were given a little piece of paper that says what animal we are, then we're blindfolded and we have to find the other chickens if we're a chicken and the other cows if we're a cow. That was so helpful! Then there's drama class, where you're suddenly speaking to a pillow and calling it mummy. Everything becomes amusing.

And that television room! I don't want to say names but there was a woman who had been in there I think 5 years or something and she was schizophrenic and I heard her say "There are poltergeists in the radiator", and I said "Now that's a great conversation opener!" One of the most famous rock stars in the world played guitar for her 60th birthday, and one of the most famous sports people presented her with something he made out of matchsticks.

All the most interesting people I think I've ever had conversations with are not celebrities; sitting in that television room, I've never had conversations like it since. That's why we keep meeting. It is really hard to wean yourself off those people because you all understand the dark side.

But now that I'm performing at some of the other Priory hospitals, the deal is - I sleep over! That's my homage to The Priory. And how frightful it is when journalists darken its reputation, because my question is: where else can somebody go when they're about to hang themselves? I just want to put that back in their court.

When I returned to being a human being, I met Mark's wife and fell in love with her and we all go on holiday together. Mark and I have one relationship when I'm well and another when I'm not. So it actually doesn't cross boundaries because the person I am when ill is hardly related to the person I am when well. So yes, I would say he saved my life. But when we're social, he's just a friend of mine.

I know Mark is a wild cookie but I don't want any staid, introverted psychiatrist giving me my medication. They've got to understand the wilderness, that's why I love him. But most of all I love The Priory. The reason I did my show is so that when I go back in again (because we all know with depression it doesn't just disappear), then I'd better get a pretty good rate!

I'm not doing all of this to help the cause of depression! I'm doing it because I'm very selfish and narcissistic. Seriously! I am doing it because God help them if I ever get depression and they dare give me a bill. Anybody at The Priory – they're going to hear about it!

It was love. When I was on tour doing a one woman show around the country, I would always make them go via The Priory, so that I could go in and smell that smell. To me it was comfort. Then they would drive me home. I can't tell you what it did for me."

Having interviewed Ruby I was keen to get to her show *Losing It*. Ruby, together with Judith Owen, a very gifted folk-jazz musician, presented a funny, poignant and thought-provoking evening. The question and answer session afterwards, when many in the audience stood up to thank Ruby for helping them come to terms with their own issues, was very moving. I had spotted Dr Collins in the front row of the stalls and enjoyed his embarrassment when Ruby forced him to take a bow.

Originally billed *Live From The Priory* and performed at the Group's hospitals all over the country, the content had changed slightly to make it attractive to a wider audience. And that of course is where Ruby Wax can use her considerable power as a popular performer to help de-stigmatise mental illness.

Ruby recently gave a talk at King's Institute of Psychiatry, when she stated her belief that people will one day look back at the early 21st century and be amazed with our collective ignorance of mental health issues. She is shocked that most people view mental illness as something that can be overcome simply with a positive attitude or 'stiff upper lip'. And while society is slowly growing more understanding of mental health conditions (the same way people hesitantly started talking about cancer 50 years ago), Ruby believes that the increasingly rapid pace of life is accelerating mental illness across the population. "Now, I can't figure out why I was ever ashamed of this." she said.

So although Ruby insisted at the end of our interview that she was not doing any of this to help the cause of clinical depression, I don't believe her.

Check out her website – www.blackdogtribe.com. It's a place where people can talk to one another about their feelings, without any reservations.

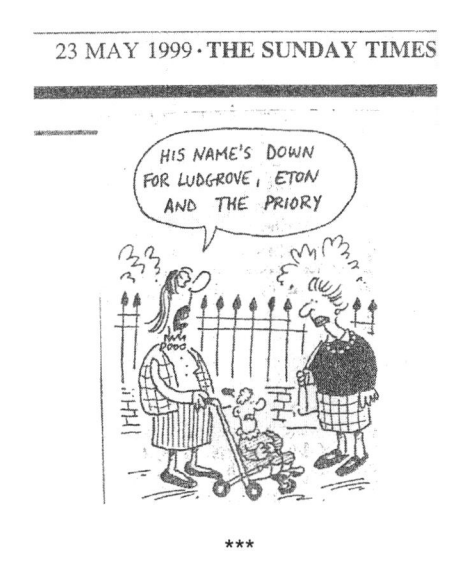

23 MAY 1999 · THE SUNDAY TIMES

His name's down for Ludgrove, Eton and the Priory

***

On occasion, if I was going into town for the evening I would leave my car at the back of the hospital and be dropped off later. One midnight, my friend Sheila drove me back to the car. We chatted for a few moments as I found my keys, and as we emerged from the car, we realised that the way out was barred by a car and a man. "That man's got a gun", hissed my fanciful friend. I had to agree that the bloke did look pretty menacing - legs akimbo, hands on hips, headlights casting a mean silhouette. Mindful of sleeping patients, Sheila whispered "Hello, we're friends", just as I twigged that it was the security guard. "Gus, it's me!" Our vigilante visibly relaxed, "Oh Dotty! Sorry! I can't be too careful at the moment."

The media would go to any lengths to bluff their way in. Just a whiff of a well-known patient and they were hiding in the shrubbery. Sometimes they would phone up, posing as a concerned relative of the alleged patient. They would pretend to be the father of so-and-so and want to speak to the doctor or some such, just to trick you into acknowledging that the person in question was indeed a patient. Politely, you would explain that you simply couldn't help them, pointing out that even if said person was a patient, you would not share that information with them or anyone else.

Unfortunately, one time it really was the father in question. I was told this later by a grim faced Dr Kelly. My heart thumped loudly and I thought *I'm fired.* Then he brightened. "Luckily" he said, "he was pleased you were so diligent."

Even worse is when you are working late and someone has sneaked into the hospital and found their way to your office. They are insisting that a certain so-and-so is an inpatient and they must see them straight away. You are aware that this person shouting and shaking their stick at you is in fact the *cause* of so-and-so's admission. You find yourself engaged in a mental game of parry and thrust. Exasperated, you are desperate for a burly male nurse to materialise and wish you had a panic button to press. Or better still, another job.

Nowadays, there is far more security at The Priory and many of the old shenanigans would be impossible. Perhaps inevitable, then, that at least one reporter has felt compelled to get herself admitted as a patient.

Nicola Gill, writing for *Cosmopolitan* actually got herself admitted under the guise of 'low self-esteem', such was her determination to find out what went on within those walls. She quickly discovers that the staff are no pushovers – two psychiatrists question her closely, the second being Dr Shur. 'Baring my soul has left me exhausted and close to tears. This is not what I expected – but it's what every patient undergoes when they arrive at The Priory.'

At her first group meeting, cross-legged on the floor with about 10 other patients, she is the only one shocked when someone dissolves into tears. Later, in the dining room, '...Kate Moss strolls in moments after me and grabs a place a couple of tables away. I'm furious to note she even manages to look stunning in hospital, wearing a skinny pink rollneck, denim skirt and knee-high boots.' After lunch, while reading the *Daily Mail*, she discovers that the fire bell that rang the night before she arrived had been caused by a fire in Kate Moss's room.

After three or four days, when she announces to Dr Shur that she's going home, he suggests she should stay longer. 'To my surprise I realise that I want to stay. When he suggests coming back for some day sessions, I agree. I've no idea what it is they've got at this place – but I can see that it definitely works.' Needless to say, when the real patients discovered that a journalist had infiltrated their group meetings, they felt betrayed.

When Rob first left rehab at Luton it seemed as though he was revelling in his sobriety. He loved being asked to speak at AA meetings, being sought after for advice, being in charge of his life. Despite my usual wariness I let myself be proud fit to burst.

But eventually we acknowledged that Rob was drinking again; he thought he now had the know-how to control it. But of course he did not and when things once again got very bad, one of his Luton buddies suggested he move to Bournemouth, which was becoming known as an established centre for addiction rehabilitation.

Initially in Bournemouth, AA meetings and sustained work for a fellow sufferer kept him on the straight and narrow. But then there were pauses in contact from him, with our own calls unanswered. It turned out that he had lost his mobile - a familiar pattern - which meant he could fall out of contact with his AA mentor and others who were treading a sober path.

Still, he got an excellent job, rented a terrific flat and met Anne, a lovely girl who was to have a very positive influence on him. He even embarked upon college studies – a Certificate in Counselling Skills. Here's an excerpt from his application to the college:

> "...Four years ago my lifestyle led me through the doors of a 3-month residential rehabilitation for drink and drug abuse. This was a vital course of action to save my life, having previously just lost my job and made a sham of any relationships I had, be it friend or family. When I emerged from this experience, awake and conscious of how I had behaved and what I had done, close friends and the family that stuck by me were really encouraged, and suggested that I would make a good counsellor. I am sure that reading this, you will be all too familiar with that almost natural human reaction. I have given this much thought, and am ready to give my all. I want to help *people* not profit margins. I want to feel good about my life and help others feel good about theirs..."

It's true that Mel and I had been warned by my Priory friends not to help Rob towards the cost of his college course – his commitment to sobriety had to come before anything else. Until he had conquered his addictions, there was no point giving him money for such a pursuit. 'He has to hit rock bottom' we were told. But he had attempted suicide at least twice (that we knew of) – would the next 'rock bottom' be the last?

It's also true that I had learned over the years to help Rob financially only when I knew exactly where the money was going. I knew all about 'tough love' from my Priory days. It had always seemed eminently sensible when the doctors and therapists warned parents and others against helping their addicted loved ones financially.

But carrying out this tough love was a tough call. I'm afraid we helped Rob towards the course anyway. We reasoned that time spent studying, writing weekly essays and being with his college peers (together with the self-knowledge he would gain along the way) was surely better than sitting alone drinking night after night.

Did we fail him? I sincerely hope not.

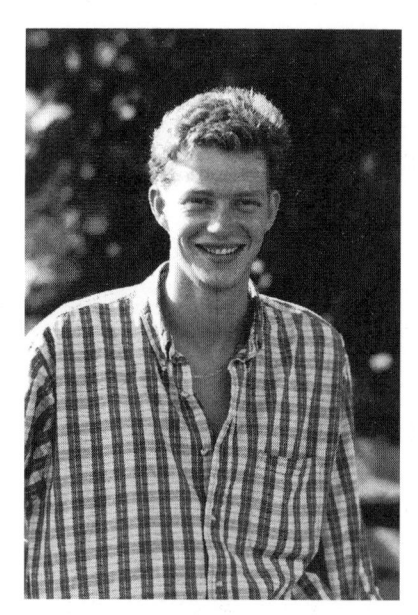

Rob, during better times

14
A Spiritual Slant

Pene Dob, Yoga Teacher
Priory Years: 1982 – 2008

> A chance meeting at a party leads to 26 years of teaching yoga at The Priory.

"Twenty six years ago I had never heard of The Priory, even though we lived so near. But we met Desmond Kelly at a party one day and we got talking and he asked what I was doing. I said yoga and he said 'Oh, would you like to come to The Priory and start teaching on Monday morning?' So I was at a party on the Saturday and on the Monday I was employed at The Priory!

Dr Kelly was the first person to introduce yoga and meditation into psychiatric medicine, and he happened to choose me to be the first yoga teacher. I think many psychiatric hospitals are doing yoga now because it's a real mind developer. Patients relate to the physical aspect of yoga, then without them even knowing, it calms their minds too. Yoga is spiritual but it isn't a religion. That's very important because you're not compromising anything. And if you are religious, it makes your own beliefs seem clearer and better.

Some of the patients were referred to me and some just came. Some of the doctors were really keen – Drs Cobb, Craggs, Islam – and of course Dr Kelly meditates himself.

I've always had really full classes – not less than 10 and sometimes up to 20 at a time. That's quite a lot, especially for a hospital where people could come and spend an hour. There were sessions on Mondays and Fridays. Then I went on to the Eating Disorders Unit (EDU), which was a third session. That class I always did in the Blue Room because it had a lovely carpet, which was more comfortable for them, being terribly thin.

I used to get letters from EDU girls saying how much they enjoyed the yoga. One of them even said she wanted to become a yoga teacher. These girls really love exercising and this was physical without actually stimulating you to lose weight – it's not running and jumping up and down but it's strenuous. And it was something they could really focus on, beyond the physical. After we had been doing an hour's yoga, we would end up with a meditation and a little bit of chanting.

Yoga teaches you to transcend whatever's getting on your nerves; to transcend it and let it be and see if you can ride on another level. That's the lovely thing about yoga. When you're under stress, you need to step out of it, and then when you go back, you're refreshed and have new insight.

I could have read their patient notes but that gives you a preconceived idea and I don't like that. I like to treat everybody as well as they present themselves and to enhance that wellness if possible. Very rarely, someone has said, oh, I can't stand this, and gone out, and I've said come back when you're feeling better – but that can happen to well people. They can come and think – *keep your brain still? How can you keep your brain still?*

I never took surnames either because when I first went there it was all very secretive – nobody wanted to brag about being in The Priory. But later on, they did. When Ruby Wax left, she told everyone: 'I learned yoga in The Priory!' I was very proud of that actually. I shouldn't be but I was! She came in two or three times and never missed a yoga class.

I remember once remarking to the secretaries that there had been a lovely girl in class that day. 'Gosh, she could be a model,' I said. They told me it was Kate Moss!

I trained as a nurse at King Edward Memorial Hospital in Ealing but nursing was really hard in those days. We did 9 nights on and 3 off. My mother, 20 years before, was doing 10 nights on and 2 off, and they had to go to their lectures after night duty. And ours wasn't a lot better all those years later. But I married my husband and he said, you're not doing that anymore.

I loved The Priory and I loved the patients. The girls were glad to see me and said I gave the place a lift. The reason for that was probably that I only did an hour and a half twice a week so I was fresh. But I think to work there continually, for long hours, it could get you down. I taught the alcoholics as well, at Galsworthy House on Kingston Hill, before it moved onto The Priory campus.

I had to step down gracefully in the end. Well, I am 69 now, and I guess the time just comes to retire, doesn't it? I've still got my church class across the road so I needn't fully retire until I'm 109!"

***

> A colleague, an eating disorders therapist, told me in the mid-Nineties, that her eye surgeon had experienced something very unusual whilst driving past The Priory. I already had thoughts of doing this book, so I said, "Oh! Do you think he'd let me interview him?" "I'm sure he would", she said. I'm abashed to admit that it was 15 years later that I contacted him. To my delight, he greeted the situation as if barely a week had passed and despite his busy life, this is what he related.

An Edwardian flashback

"About 25 years ago I used to take a short-cut through Richmond Park on my way to Oxford from Wimbledon, before the M40 was built. The wall concerned in my story faces the Roehampton Club golf course across the road, along which I was driving alone in the car. I have never seen the other side of this wall.

What I saw was a young woman walking along by the wall in the middle of a bright sunny day. Her apparel was the most striking feature and were it not for that I probably would not have noticed anything unusual. The girl's appearance made me think at first that she was going to a fancy dress party. She wore a long skirt and blouse in the manner of an Edwardian working woman with a flat-brimmed straw hat. The hatband seemed to be decorated with something, perhaps foliage, flowers or fruit. She was not in the slightest ghostly. I was so impressed with the outfit that I looked round as I drove past. It was only then that I was taken aback by what I had observed because she was nowhere to be seen!

I actually stopped the car and walked the full length of the wall in both directions, as well as looking across the road onto the golf course. She was still nowhere to be seen and I was unable to find any gate or opening through which she might have left the footpath in the few seconds between my seeing her and passing by in the car.

Other than family, I hadn't mentioned this to anyone until I met someone years later who worked in The Priory, so felt tempted to enquire whether anyone else there had shared my experience.

There must be a plausible if obscure cause and probably such experiences are more commonplace than we think. It hasn't altered my generally sceptical attitude to the supernatural. Over the years, though, I have met other highly objective people who have recounted similarly odd happenings. I shall be very interested if anyone else has shared this sort of Priory experience."

Mr John L Hungerford, Consultant Ophthalmologist

15
The Importance of Being Earnie

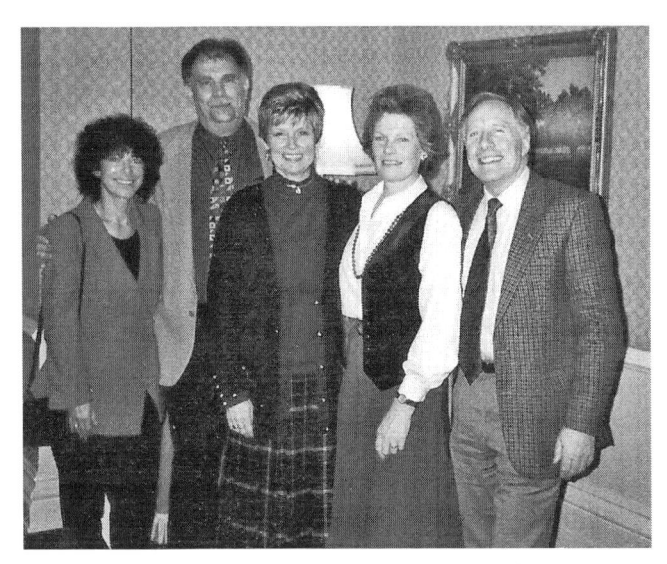

Left to right: Chris Ball, Earnie & Paula Larsen, Angela & Desmond Kelly

Earnie Larsen burst upon The Priory scene from Minneapolis, with an abundance of energy and enthusiasm. If the doctors or therapists had any reticence about him initially, they were soon won over by his earthy, humorous approach to the most challenging of human situations. Earnie broadened The Priory's therapeutic horizons.

"I was ordained a Catholic priest in 1965. My family background was always heavy on 'stick up for your people' and 'leave the world better than you found it.' Since my family tree was full of alcoholics and folks with mental problems they naturally became my people The 'leave the world better than you found it' was just another way of saying, 'do service work'. So all in all I guess it's no surprise that once I resigned the priesthood in 1978, I would move into working with alcoholics and people with dual-diagnosis issues.

I wrote my first book in 1967. I didn't intend it to be a book. At the time I was stationed at an inner city parish in St Louis, Missouri. The religious text book we had was written for middle class white kids. The book had nothing to do with the culture and situation of the kids I was working with. So I drew up an outline of what I wanted to teach the next year.

The order I belonged to had a publishing arm. They took the book and put it out in book form called 'Good Old Plastic Jesus'. It took off and eventually sold over a quarter million copies. So that got me both writing and speaking at many religious education conventions and 12-step gatherings. Here it is 40 years later and I've pretty much kept doing the same thing: books, films and conventions.

My wife Paula and I first went to The Priory in January 1995. We were thrilled to get an invitation and the prime mover behind the offer was Dr Kelly. For some reason he knew of my work and thought it might be helpful to the program at The Priory.

My first impression of Roehampton was "My gosh: it's a palace!" But consistently over the years as we visited The Priory what stood out more than anything was the competent and loving staff. We've visited many treatment facilities and none ever had a more committed, caring staff.

The quality of the staff always ultimately reflects the quality of the leadership. In this regard, I can't say enough about the leadership shown by Dr Kelly. There aren't many people who rise to the position of authority attained by Dr Kelly who remain as humble, grateful and open to learn anything that may better his program than he. If I had a hall of fame of most memorable people I've met along the way, Dr Kelly would certainly be there in a place of honor.

An interesting event – at least to me – was an evening presentation hosted by The Priory at the Royal Society of Medicine, No.1 Wimpole Street. Many in attendance were in black tie, the women in gowns. I had never been in a situation like that before and wondered how an American cowboy would come across to such a learned and formal audience. I guess it went well. No one booed or threw anything.

During the mixing with people after the program, a man came up wearing a heavy white sweater, no suit coat or formal attire. He shook my hand and said, 'Hello, my name is Eric. I want to thank you for tonight. Your books have helped me in my recovery.' I thanked him and basically that was that.

It was only later I learned he was the world famous rock star, Eric Clapton. He was just another bloke in recovery, getting by the best he could.

Some time later, Eric came to Minneapolis, where Paula and I live, to do a concert. He called and we got together for breakfast at the downtown hotel where he was staying. The woman who waited on us obviously recognised Mr Clapton. As we got ready to leave she cleared her throat and hesitantly said to him, 'My name is Nancy. I have nine months clean today. I want to thank you for making it acceptable to be in recovery.' Eric turned in his chair to look her full in the face, took her hand, and told her how proud he was of her. He told her the first thing he does whenever he gets to a different city is look up where a meeting is, because 'we are all in the same boat.' He made her feel ten foot tall. For that moment she was the only person in the room. She had his full attention. [Eric Clapton later named one of the units at Crossroads, his addictions hospital in Antigua, after Earnie Larsen].

Another interesting event was an afternoon program for family physicians we did at The Priory. Many people on both sides of the pond told me to not expect 'reserved Englishmen' to share their experience in the same way Americans do. But a key element of everything I know and do in my presentations is ask 'hard questions'. By that I mean personal questions that lead to the core issues of addiction and recovery. So I thought it would be interesting to see how the physicians responded to the only way I know how to teach.

I need not have worried. The sharing was loud, long and intense. Several of the staff later told me, 'I never would have believed it!'

We met and became friends with many staff members at The Priory and were blessed to do an intensive staff training for our Life Management Program. We stayed in contact with several members of that training for years.

Dr Kelly sets the tone for The Priory and is, say those who know him well, able to calm an agitated person by talking to them quietly for a minute or so. He practises what he preaches: he meditates every day and jogs in Richmond Park, though not after dark, 'in case I disturb the deer.' Not least, he insists on time out. When I saw him last he was off to Cardiff to watch the rugby.

Paula and I consider our contact with The Priory and the deep friendships we formed there as one of the highest highlights of our careers. We will be forever thankful that Dr Kelly invited us into The Priory family."

During the time of putting this book together, I read *You Don't Have To Be Famous To Have Manic Depression* by Dr Tony Hughes and Jeremy Thomas. I was romping through at a great pace but sat up straight when, in one of the dialogues between the two authors, Jeremy said:

> "I went and saw DK at the Priory Hospital in Roehampton again and said I needed a 100,000 mile service and some Prozac. He asked me why I wanted the Prozac. I told him I'd discovered one or two of my more cheerful friends had been taking it for some time and thought to myself, *Well, no wonder they were so bloody cheerful!* DK said to me, 'Look, you cannot take anything like Prozac, because it might make you manic.'
>
> He said, 'You've got to keep going.' He suggested reading two books that he knew were very helpful for people with a dual diagnosis of manic depression and alcoholism and all that stuff. I got the books and thought, *Oh my God, I'm turning into a self-help twat.*"

But Jeremy found the books extremely helpful. They were *Believing in Myself* (Earnie Larsen and Carol Hegarty), and *Stage II Recovery: Life Beyond Addiction* (Earnie Larsen).

Jeremy is a huge admirer of Earnie's work and in a recent email to me, he said:

> "I think he made an original, practical and immensely insightful contribution to people recovering from depressive and addictive illnesses. Top top geezer."

Earnie died on January 11, 2011, at the age of 71. Less than 48 hours before, he had given a lecture to a crowd of more than 500, most of whom would have known that his battle with pancreatic cancer was all but over.

His final book *Now That You're Sober* came out in 2010. In it he described being a grateful member of the Twelve Step family since 1966. He had written more than sixty recovery and spirituality books and authored dozens of DVDs and CD programmes in America during that time.

I believe that the importance of being Earnie was that he personified his family's moral code to leave the world better than you found it, and his books live on to continue his work.

16
Princess Diana and The Priory

A highlight of the tenth year of The Priory Hospitals Group (PHG) was an invitation to participate in a Royal seminar on community care and mental health issues. The idea to bring together the public, voluntary and private sectors came from Turning Point, the largest charity in the UK dealing with drink, drugs and mental health problems. And the idea received the approval of their Patron, Her Royal Highness the Princess of Wales.

In October 1990 St Augustine's Hospital in Chartham Canterbury, played host to a visit by the Princess and provided the venue for the seminar. The hospital, a typically large mental institution, was in the process of moving patients into the community. It had only a fraction of the original number of patients remaining and the Princess managed to fit in visits to three wards. The patients and staff were thrilled. The visit was a real morale booster during the difficult final phase of the closure programme. The Priory staff had been briefed: "She is tall, a fast walker and very much brighter than the media gives her credit for."

At 10.30am the air was thick with excitement as the Royal party arrived by helicopter. The Princess of Wales was escorted by the Deputy Lieutenant of Kent from the landing site just in front of St Augustine's Hospital. As Chairman of PHG, Desmond Kelly's task was to accompany her around the wards and he was immediately struck by the profound effect she had on people.

When one elderly lady was introduced, the Princess asked 'How are you today?' The lady replied, 'I'm very worried, you see it's my belt.' The Princess threw open the tartan jacket she was wearing and showed the surprised lady the safety pin in her own skirt, demonstrating what she did to make herself more comfortable. 'Nobody will know!' she said. The patient lit up like a Christmas tree.

In June 1993 PHG was honoured by the first Royal visit to one of its hospitals - Grovelands Priory – where Princess Diana made the keynote address at a seminar called 'Women and Mental Health – Counting the Cost of Caring'. Jean Kilshaw, PHG's Communications Consultant, made this happen for The Priory by working with Turning Point again, as in 1990.

With the Princess of Wales there the media were out in force. Also speaking were Dr Fiona Caldicott, Dean, and first woman President-Elect of the Royal College of Psychiatrists, and Dr Rachel Jenkins, Principal Medical Officer for Mental Health at the Department of Health. Miss Libby Purves, Journalist and Broadcaster, took the Chair, and Dr Miriam Stoppard, writer and broadcaster, also contributed.

Inside The Priory

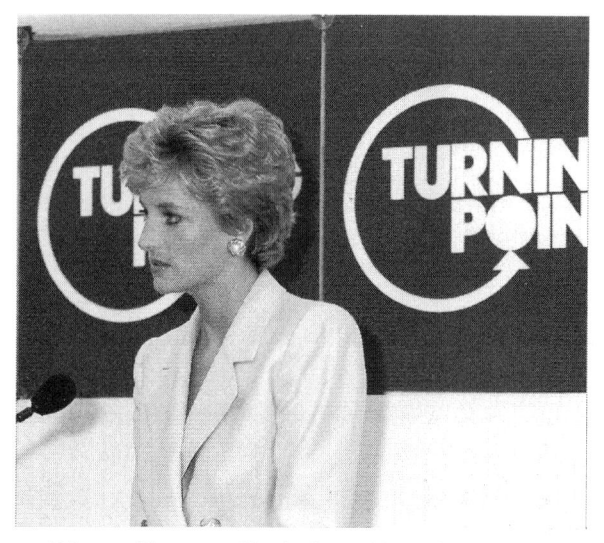

Princess Diana speaking in June 1993 at Grovelands Priory

In her book *Diana*, the historian and biographer Sarah Bradford explains that the Princess was determined to be seen as a professional on these occasions and had employed a voice coach, Peter Settelen, to teach her voice techniques to improve her public speaking.

> "A visit to Great Ormond Street Hospital, where she learned more about a subject close to her – eating disorders in young women – led to her speech in Kensington Town Hall in April 1993 which was widely publicised and brought eating disorders to the top of the public agenda. Diana was delighted with the speech, not only because Settelen had taught her how to express emotion in public speaking (too much so in the view of Diana's aides) but because she had come close to expressing her personal experience and suffering. As patron of the charity Turning Point, she spoke at a conference in June 1993 about the need for support of mentally ill women. The conference was chaired by Libby Purves who said, 'The Princess is one of us, a wife, a mother, a daughter who has known problems in her own life and who has courageously used these experiences to comfort other people.' It did not escape the general public that no other member of the Royal Family would have addressed personal issues in such a way."

Here are excerpts from Princess Diana's address at Grovelands Priory:

> "Whatever life throws at them – women will always cope. On call 24 hours a day, seven days a week, whether their children are sick, their husbands out of work or their parents are old and frail and need attending – they will cope.
>
> "Frequently they will attempt to survive it alone, falling 'help-lessly'

into a deeper and darker depression as they feel more and more trapped by the life they are leading.

"Perhaps we need to look more closely at the cause of the illness rather than attempt to suppress it. To accept that putting a lid on powerful feelings and emotions cannot be the healthy option. That to offer women the opportunity to explain their predicament sooner could be a far more effective use of resources, rather than wait until their strength to survive has been sapped.

"As long as the real reasons for their problems go unnoticed and unattended they will continue to pass on to the next generation their 'dis-ability'.

"If we as a society continue to disable women, by encouraging them to believe they should only do things that are thought to benefit their family even if these women are 'damaged' in the process; if they feel they never have the right to do anything that is just for themselves; if they feel they must sacrifice everything for their loved ones even at the cost of their health, their inner strength and their own self-worth; they will live only in the shadow of others and their mental health will surely suffer. But if we can help to give them back their right to fulfil their own potential and to share that with their family, children or friends, maybe fewer women would find themselves living a life that is bleak beyond belief.

"Each person is born with very individual qualities and potential. We as a society owe it to women to create a truly supportive environment in which they too can grow and move forward. But if we are to help the quiet private desperate lives lived behind closed doors by so many women, they need to know for certain they are not alone – that real support and understanding is there for them.

"I hope this conference will help us to understand the needs of women more clearly and that you will find a way of reaching them more effectively and help to give them back their rightful, mentally healthy life."

The Princess's address achieved phenomenal media coverage. It was broadcast on *Woman's Hour* and even made the American press. Turning Point had never experienced anything like it. The event was a front page story and many papers reproduced the speech in full.

The reaction was extremely favourable, with the content and delivery described as "powerful", "poignant", eloquent", "far-reaching", "concerned" and "controversial". The over-riding view was that it had come from the heart.

This was a time when The Roehampton Priory and the Group as a whole were building bridges with the Royal College of Psychiatrists and helping the Defeat Depression Campaign.

Inside The Priory

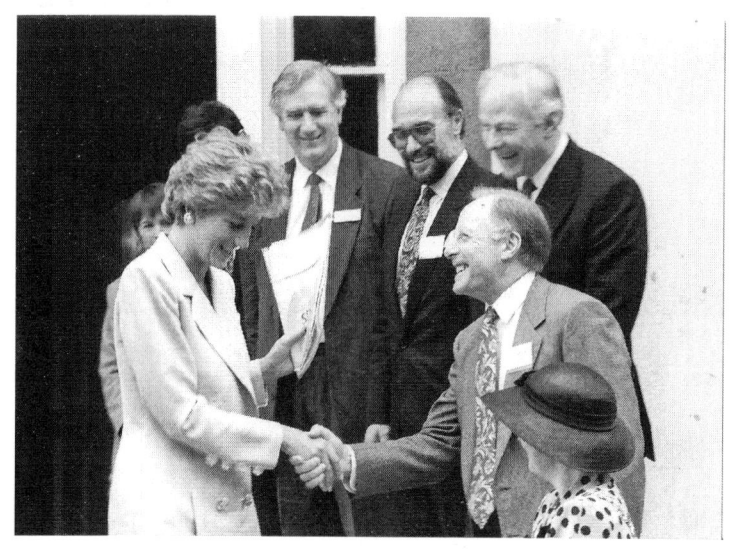

"Don't you dare fall down these steps!"

The Priory was also enjoying strong links with St George's Hospital in Tooting. For several years there had been an outpatient bulimia clinic at The Priory, run in collaboration with St George's under the auspices of Professor Hubert Lacey. The Clinic's Senior Registrar, who was involved with the treatment programme, was funded by The Priory Research Fellowship. With demand for eating disorder treatment in the NHS in London outstripping supply, the existence of The Priory's Clinic filled an important gap in service provision.

St George's had a great interest in eating disorders, thanks to the influence of Professors Arthur Crisp and Hubert Lacey. The Priory was fortunate to have Dr Peter Rowan who had set up and was running the Eating Disorders Unit. He had been a colleague of Desmond Kelly at St George's before moving to The Priory.

In 1997 the anorexic girls at The Priory wrote to Princess Diana asking if she would come to pay them an unofficial visit. To their delight, she said yes. Her visit was a closely kept secret; there was to be no media involvement and the Medical Director and Priory staff were not involved. It was strictly between the patients and Princess Diana.

Her visit was an outstanding success. The Princess spoke of her experience first and then everyone joined in. The patients were bubbling over with enthusiasm and gratitude.

Dr Peter Rowan told me some years later:

> "I deliberately didn't get involved in Princess Diana's visit, although I was running the unit when she came. It was the patients

themselves who had asked her to come. The patients loved it and the feedback afterwards was that it helped them feel better about themselves and since that's a very fundamental issue in anorexia, no doubt it was helpful.

It was the fact that Princess Di felt they were important enough to actually take the trouble to be there, all that non-verbal communication and warmth was actually what it was about, much more than anything that was actually said. It was the feeling that she managed to give people – that they were valuable and important to her.

She was such an icon that when she did that it had a pretty powerful impact. Particularly on them because they were fragile, had low self-esteem and low sense of self-worth and suddenly you get somebody like that coming round who has been through it."

Priory cleaner, Clara Guagueta, has a cherished memory about Princess Diana at The Priory:

"I remember a friend of Princess Diana was in the hospital and he and I used to chat. One day he whispered: 'Tomorrow, Princess Diana is coming at 3pm, so if you want to see her she will come in to Reception.' I said 'Thank you very much!' Next afternoon I went to my room and changed into jeans and a nice jumper. Patrick was working at Reception – what a gentleman. Mail for the staff was kept behind the desk. I said, 'Patrick I want to see a very important letter from Colombia.' He Said 'Clara, please, no, not now.' The area had been cleared because she was coming but I pretended not to notice a thing. I said 'Oh please, please.' And just then Princess Diana came in. I was so excited! I said: 'Oh Princess Diana! How are you?' She said 'Hello, how are you?' And then I introduced Patrick! I was so emotional. I went to my room and said 'Thank you God! Thank you, thank you.' I phoned my parents in Colombia, who said I was crazy. They didn't even know who Princess Diana was! When she died it was like losing a member of the family. I went to all the places where people were gathering and spent nearly £100 on flowers. I was mad with grief."

17
Going Public: Priory within the community

> "Community is an important word in the vocabulary of the staff at The Priory and their aim is to make this historic hospital as much a part of the fabric of its south London community as possible."
>
> *Dr Desmond Kelly, Nursing Focus, September 1982*

The Priory (indeed the whole Group) became active in the community and supported charities concerned with the Group's key interests, particularly mental health. Depression initiatives, such as the Defeat Depression Campaign – a joint venture between the Royal College of Psychiatrists and the Royal College of General Practitioners – was heavily promoted and supported, both practically and financially by The Priory.

Here are just a few of the other ways it became involved in the community.

Seminars

The Priory seminars were mighty popular with general practitioners, psychiatrists and therapists. This was probably down to the mix of excellent speakers, a delicious buffet lunch, and tea with networking and gossip to follow.

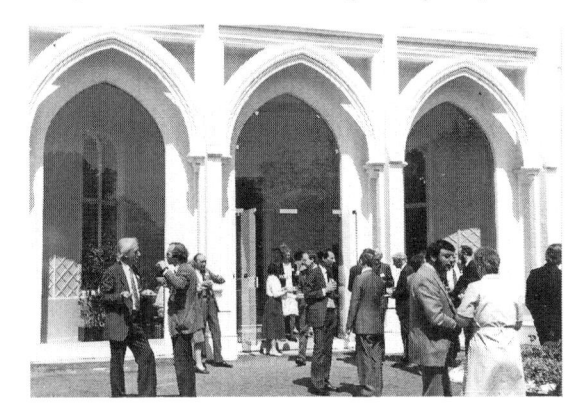

For the real enthusiast of seminars, see the listing at the end of the book.

Dr Ralph Burton, Fitznells Manor General Practice

> A retired GP, Dr Burton looks back on how the Roehampton Priory influenced his own practice, one of the first to join the Primary Care Trust system.

"GP fund holding was an initiative of the Conservative Government when Ken Clarke was Minister for Health in 1991. It was killed in name by political forces in 1998, although the concept could still be seen in other initiatives and if you were clever enough in managing the system, you were able to retain most of the gains.

In the beginning we were a partnership of four, practising at Fitznells Manor in Ewell, Surrey. There was not an identified element for mental health but we took the view that it was an essential part of a medical service and that we should use our budget to improve what was, at that time, an almost non-existent service from secondary care. Mental health was under the supposed direction of the acute service but through a mixture of neglect and attrition they had virtually no service to offer when we required specialist input.

The Priory had a high reputation in the private sector and the service given to patients who could afford it was second to none. It contrasted starkly with the service provided by the NHS at that time. Dr Kelly was clearly identified as the figurehead at The Priory and most of us had previous experience of his services, in that he had become the foremost provider of education in all things psychiatric. This attracted us by a combination of high quality education and superb catering – a winning combination for any GP.

We thought how wonderful it would be if only we could obtain some of this quality of service for our NHS patients. I didn't think we had much hope of success and initially approached Dr Kelly with the idea of purchasing some slots for our patients at The Priory, but it became clear that our money would not go very far and we would only be able to benefit a few.

It was Dr Kelly who came up with the offer that he would be willing to pilot a process whereby he would visit Fitznells on a regular basis, to give a 'one off' input into cases we were stuck with, to see if he could break the impasse, and then hand them on (usually with a plan) to ongoing care within the Practice.

So it was that Dr Kelly's monthly trips to Fitznells started and continued right up until his retirement. During this time he must have seen over 500 of our patients and in many cases produced a major breakthrough in their care. Many patients remembered their consultation with Dr Kelly as a turning point in their lives. He also taught many of our trainees, as well as introducing large numbers of medical students to the wonders of managing psychiatric problems in primary care.

But here's an anecdote to keep things in perspective. Hettie was a single, late middle-aged woman living with her brother and his wife (saints both), who seemed somehow to get into almost every Monday morning surgery. She was consumed by anxiety but as far as I could tell had no physical basis for her many complaints. This was before MRI scanners but she had received every test up to that point and all were normal. I referred her to Dr Kelly although her belief was that 'they should cut me open and have a look inside'.

After seeing Dr Kelly she still appeared in my surgery the following Monday:

RB: How are you feeling Hettie?
HL: Terrible. I'm so worried.
RB: But you have just seen our specialist, Dr Kelly. What did he say?
HL: He told me not to worry.
RB: Then why can't you accept that?
HL: He's a doctor isn't he? What's he going to say: 'Worry?' "

GROW

Desmond Kelly's championing of the self-help movement has been described as 'avant-garde'. He took every opportunity to stress the important part that self-help groups have to play in the management of psychological illness, even encouraging their formation and regular meetings at The Priory itself. And as Chairman of the British National Committee for the Prevention and Treatment of Depression, he got together with Richard France to edit *A Practical Handbook for the Treatment of Depression* published in 1987. Designed as a guide for physicians, the book paved the way for the introduction of GROW in England.

A patient, Christine Ward, explains:

> "In the autumn of 1983, I spent three weeks at The Priory. My treatment consisted of administering drugs and a short course of ECT (I was lucky enough to respond well to this) but depression had been a problem for me over a ten year period and I asked Dr Kelly if there was anything I could do to avoid it in future.
>
> Around the time of me leaving, Dr Kelly heard of a mental health self-help organisation called GROW, in Ireland. Father Donal Spring agreed to come over and lead a small 'taster' group.
>
> The outcome was that I was very impressed by the group method and Dr Kelly asked if I would like to run a GROW group at The Priory.
>
> Although GROW was new to us, it already existed in Australia (its birthplace), New Zealand, Ireland, Illinois, Canada and Mauritius. GROW's programme of personal growth, caring and sharing, developed from the findings of former mental health sufferers in the course of rebuilding their lives after breakdown.
>
> The group was started by Con Keogh [Father Cornelius Keogh, an Australian Roman Catholic priest], after his own personal breakdown in 1957. At that time, the only other self-help organisation was AA. He saw the value of the 12-step system and included it in the first groups, which were called Recovery. Soon, however, the groups were called GROW in order to meet the increasing demand for the groups' services in prevention as well as rehabilitation."

International Stress Management Association

Desmond Kelly first met Joe Macdonald Wallace, a Health Education Consultant, at the University of Sussex in 1983. Joe founded a voluntary, non-profit health agency – International Stress and Tension Control Society (as it was then called) and asked if DK would help form a branch at The Priory Hospital. Joe was delighted when it became a very strong branch, and The Priory became, in effect, the head office.

In September 1998, at the Third International Congress on Stress Management, hosted by the University of Edinburgh, Desmond was elected International President of the Society and its influence grew over the next few years.

Author and journalist Stephen Pile came to Edinburgh for the conference and he gave a great description of Joe in his article *Relax - I just can't stress that enough* in the *Sunday Times* on 4 September 1988.

> "The conference was organised by the cherubic Joe Macdonald Wallace, who ought to have been a stretcher case. Every time you saw Joe he was surrounded by tall Germans who had lost their luggage, or on the phone to three speakers cancelling at the last minute, or striding around holding four conversations at once. Throughout he remained calm, as befits the author of *Stress: a Practical Guide to Coping*."

Bemused by the 100 talks and workshops on offer, Stephen Pile realised that everybody on the planet is stressed to the eyeballs.

> "...Stress in pregnancy, the menopause and bereavement, stress in students, the homesick, Finnish public health administrators, South African executives, motoring stress and stress in Hamburg dentists."

The most helpful session for him was held by Laura Mitchell (of the Mitchell Method) whose floor exercises had him on his feet again feeling better than he had for years.

Letter to my sister Susan, 6/11/88

> "...The stress congress in Edinburgh was fun. I knew I should attend some lectures and workshops but was overwhelmed by the huge choice, with 23 nations represented.
>
> It was all very well organised so nothing to worry about for me except that I found myself pursued by two professors; a Russian and a Bulgarian. The Bulgarian had a limp, an advantage for the Russian. When a party of us went on a coach tour of the Trossachs, the Russian sat next to me. I dozed off three times as it was raining and I couldn't see much. He took to waking me up by stroking my leg. The first time I thought it was a mistake – maybe he'd been asleep too and momentarily thought I was someone else. The second and third times, I knew. I didn't want to antagonise him, especially as Dr Kelly says he is the most

influential psychiatrist in the USSR, so I smiled sweetly as I prised his fingers from my knee.

At Loch Lomond he and the Bulgarian asked me to take a photo of them together. The Bulgarian said the photo should be called 'The Optimist and the Pessimist'. The Russian took me aside and whispered, "My friend, he is the optimist during the day. But me, I am the optimist at night." This gave me pause for thought, since I knew his room was near mine back at the campus. That evening, I quietly absented myself from the entertainment and sprinted down the corridors to evade nocturnal Slavic optimism. As I ran, I wished I had paid more attention to the lecture given by the very same Russian that morning – 'Neurophysiological Mechanisms of Behaviour Self-Regulation during Emotional Stress in Animals.'

Four years later, in 1992, the Pierre et Marie Curie University in Paris hosted the Fourth International Conference. It was at the end of this conference that Desmond Kelly retired from the Presidency. ISMA had become an important health promotion agency in a dozen countries and a life saver in many languages.

Neuromapping

In 1988, the Group made a major investment at The Roehampton Priory when it installed a brain mapper. The move was part of Dr Kelly's strategy to keep The Priory Hospitals Group (PHG) at the forefront of the private psychiatric sector. An internationally known Clinical Neurophysiologist, Dr Peter Fenwick, from the Maudsley Hospital, came on board as Director of Neurophysiology Services.

In the spring of 1990 Priory Hospitals Group News (written and edited by the Communications Officer Jean Kilshaw) announced:

"The usefulness of the brain mapper in patients with epilepsy has led to a collaboration between The Priory Hospital, Roehampton, and the Oxford Health Authority. The latter does not have the facilities to investigate patients in this way and so The Priory offered to provide a full neurophysiological assessment service for the NHS patients."

The Priory was the only private psychiatric hospital with a brain mapper and it was important to make sure its potential was fully realised. The arrangement with Oxford brought the two together in the best interests of patients.

The brain mapper had important applications in psychiatry, not least because it could monitor the response of the brain to a stimulus. Brainwave activity was converted into brain maps, which enabled brain function to be studied – a considerable asset in the diagnosis of neurological disorders such as epilepsy and psychiatric illness.

Another service the brain mapper enabled The Priory to offer was something very rare in the UK at the time – sleep assessment. As PHG News described:

> "The Priory Hospital is now able to offer a full sleep pathology and diagnostic service. The prescribing of hypnotics without prior investigation is no longer seen as the answer to even 'routine' sleep problems. Rather, thorough assessment of the underlying mechanisms is the basis for sound therapeutic decisions.
>
> Management may not require the use of drugs at all but readjustments of sleep/wake behaviour. The brain mapper can help re-set the body clock and turn owls into larks. Many people are late to bed and late to rise. This is fine for the individual only if his or her lifestyle and occupation permit. For the majority they do not. In the sleep laboratory the individual can be monitored and the sleep/wake times adjusted by two hours every day until they are back with the rest of us. And there they stay. A fascinating use of this new 'window' on the brain."

The Seven Ages of Woman Symposium

A highlight of The Priory's outreach activities took place in September 1991 when PHG held a symposium at The Royal College of Physicians in London.

The Chairperson for the morning session was Dr Fiona Caldicott, Dean of The Royal College of Psychiatrists, who congratulated The Priory Hospitals Group on their imaginative choice of subject for the symposium, which encompassed important issues affecting various stages of a girl's life, from childhood through to the later years. Addressing the general practitioners in the audience, she emphasised the importance of the link between GPs and psychiatrists in developing community services for the psychiatrically ill. Speakers included Dr Sara McCluskey, a Priory Research Fellow, who presented her findings about abnormal eating behaviour and its associations with changes in the ovary. At the end of the day Dr Caldicott summed up by saying that the papers had been "outstanding examples of the contribution of psychiatric research to patient care."

Putney Samaritans

As one of The Priory's outreach efforts, Dr Kelly became Honorary Psychiatrist to the Putney Samaritans group. A major objective of The Priory was to keep people safe and prevent suicides and he worked with Ernest Spry of the Putney branch to offer local help.

Ernest Spry very kindly arranged for me to undergo training to become a Samaritan. He knew I had no intention of becoming a Samaritan (particularly when working at The Priory) but he was aware of the unpredictable nature of my job, including phone calls from despairing patients.

The training was thought-provoking, to say the least, and the 'Sams' running the sessions were delightful. I finished that course with huge admiration for their patience, tolerance and humanity. I also did a foundation year in 'person-centred' counselling at the Metanoia Trust whilst working at The Priory. It was utterly fascinating but sufficient to convince me that I didn't have the right make-up to be a counsellor.

For all psychiatrists, a patient's suicide is the ultimate failure. On the eve of his retirement, DK was interviewed by Margarette Driscoll of *The Sunday Times* and was able to tell her that mercifully few patients of his had taken their own lives. One patient had thrown himself from a seventh-floor balcony only to land in a skip, breaking his wrist. Another got lost on the way to Beachy Head. "There is only so much a psychiatrist can do. Sometimes you must rely on divine providence," he said.

18
Time Out

I imagine that right back to Dr William Wood's time, staff at The Priory found ways to take time out together, as a counter-balance to the rigours of their work and as a way of getting to know each other in a relaxed way.

We know the staff put on productions during Erich Herrmann's time (from the 1950s onwards) but there is little record of this, other than a note his wife Joyce wrote me.

> "My first encounter with The Priory was when after a staff meeting it was decided that a play should be put on. Both staff and patients should be involved. Erich was full of excitement when he arrived home. The cast had been selected, Erich was the sound and lighting engineer, and he had volunteered my services to be the make-up artist! The first play was *A Midsummer Night's Dream*. The 'actors' were staff, their children, and patients."

This was during Dr Forsyth's reign. He had a penchant for amateur dramatics and one Christmas he decided that staff and patients should mount a production of Scrooge at short notice. Albert Stickland, the clerk of works, was dragooned into playing Scrooge, scrambling about in a nightshirt on an upturned table, draped to resemble a four poster. None of the 'actors' were given time to learn their lines so Dr Forsyth stalked about the stage bellowing promptings.

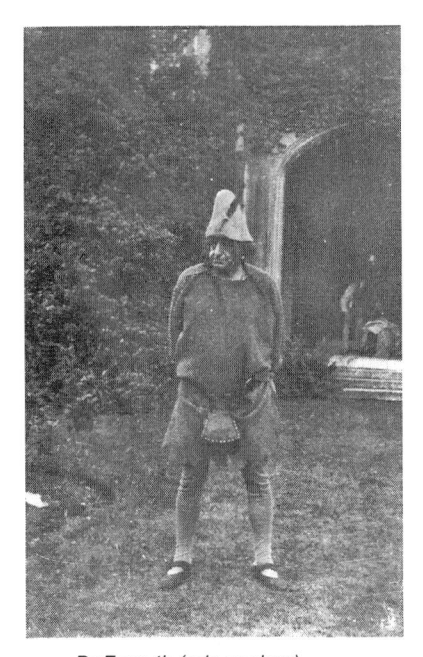

Dr Forsyth (role unclear)

Inspired by this dramatic success, Dr Forsyth founded The Priory Players, who staged occasional plays, including *A Midsummer Night's Dream*, in which he cast himself as Bottom.

At New Year there would be a lavish fancy dress party for all the staff, during which Dr Forsyth would make it his business to get to know his more comely female employees.

Fast forward a few years and an example of relaxing with colleagues in the 1980s and '90s, was the Visiting Consultants Dinner. An annual feast, the dinners were a form of thank you to VCs by the full-time Consultants, for their support. Up to 50 shrinks would attend, all in the best of humour and at their most charming. The service was impeccable, with delectable food and wine and Pedro the head waiter was in his element.

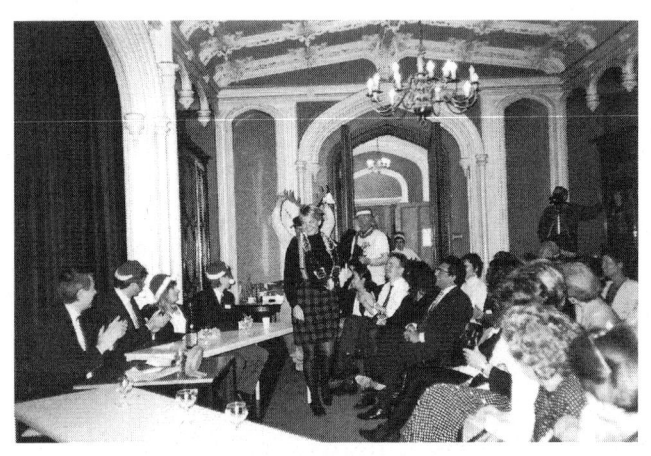

A Call My Bluff team makes a festive entrance

In 1992, Head Office decided that an 'outward bound' course would be good for Priory management and so in October a group of us set off for the depths of rural Wales. We were instructed to take at least three complete changes of old, warm clothes and be prepared to get dirty and wet. Walking boots, waterproofs and a good torch were also essential kit. We feared the worst.

Shortly after arrival at a rustic hostel we embarked on our first exercise: find lunch. We were split into groups and armed with ordnance survey maps, which we took turns in trying to decipher. My group eventually found lunch, courtesy of a bearded walker and his collie dog who tipped us the wink about a table of goodies nearby. It was an action-packed weekend, at times exhilarating and at times plain scary.

One exercise involved five of us and was called 'Blindfold Walk'. Unsurprisingly, we were blindfolded, issued with helmets and driven we knew not where. Once we had fallen out of the mini-van, our brief was to keep hold of each other at all times. A senior male nurse called Mac led and I was close behind. We travelled a tortuous path, up and down steep slippery slopes with close vegetation on one side and nothingness sensed on the other. All we could do was hold on, communicate, and trust each other. When we were shown where we'd been afterwards, we were jolly glad for the blindfolds.

As a result of that long weekend, one or two colleagues who had hitherto seemed a touch frivolous, turned out to have useful strengths. We all had to take challenges back and mine (as work comes easier than play), was to set up a Fun Committee. I became the 'Mistress of Fun'. Our committee went on to dream up all sorts of events and aside from our own immense enjoyment, it really did seem to have a positive impact on staff morale.

A highlight for the Fun Committee came in October 1995, when we staged The Priory's version of *Blind Date*. We managed to unearth a good-looking unattached young man, who agreed to play along. I believe he was very impressed with the three genuine single beauties jostling for his favours – Moe, Pippa and Kirsty (Chairman's PA, a Psychiatrist, and Head of Occupational Therapy, respectively).

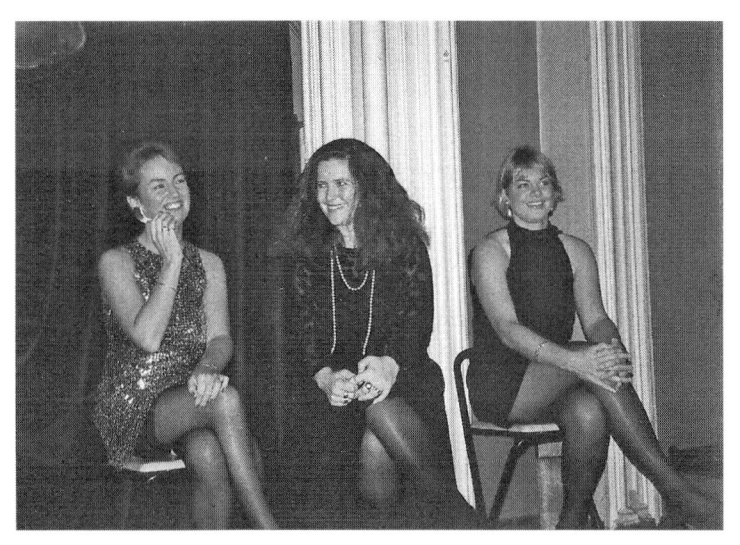

Moe, Pippa and Kirsty

Our second trio of contenders were nervously anticipated by a big-hearted young man from Head Office. He couldn't believe his pluck (pun intended) when they minced around the screen towards him, to the huge delight of the audience.

I'm not sure whether any of the inpatients at the time caught sight of their psychiatrists in drag and how that might have affected their recovery but we of the Fun Committee made sure that our special ladies were well prepared for performance. Their dressing room was abuzz with make-up tips and raucous banter as their hair and manicure artistes (aka Virginia and Dianne, Pharmacist and Admissions Manager), got creative. Dr Shur was being a diva about his nails; Dr King-Lewis was looking up Dr Collins's skirt (we never knew why) and Dr Collins gradually assumed the persona of his alter ego, Lady Letitia. He recalls the event:

> "People commented that I seemed to be rather preoccupied with getting my makeup right, as *if* it were something I might have loved! Of course this was the first time for me. We had Chris Prestwood who was in charge of the Eating Disorders Unit as Cilla; Peter King-Lewis, a GP trainee at the time and now a private GP, dressed up as Matron, and Dr Shur was a drag queen (the South African version of Dame Edna Everage). And I was Lady Letitia Straddling-Cox.
>
> That event was completely indicative of the atmosphere of the place, and it was important that we had a Fun Committee. Although it's a bit of a cliché, having the consultants participate at that level was really good and gets everyone to feel part of it. It's a real shame that it's no longer done."

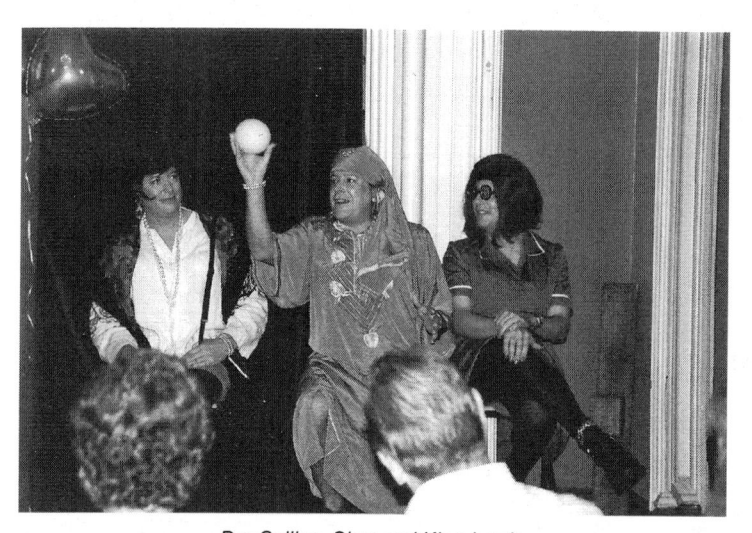

Drs Collins, Shur and King-Lewis

And Dr Shur:

> "The idea of Mark Collins, Peter King-Lewis and me dressing up as women was good because it cut us down to size if you like! I went to a shop in Brixton and bought a beautiful dress from Ghana. I've still got it but I should tell you on record that I only wore it that once! I really enjoyed dressing up as a woman. You know the fascinating thing was that people reacted to me as if I *was* a woman, pinching my bottom and flirting with me, in a way which was very surprising and quite shocking. For a second I began to see what it must be like for a woman. But it was great fun, particularly when I was chosen for a date!

"These occasions were quite unique I think. I don't know of another hospital that did things like this. It was very good for morale. When you left Dotty, they tried to reconstitute it but it never really came off for some reason. Fortunately, it was recorded on video. Taking part in *Blind Date* will always be one of my happiest memories of The Priory."

By the time I left, two years before DK would retire, I sensed that it was now or never. I had been offered a job with a charity guru and, after all, I had been at The Priory for more than a third of my life. It did seem a touch reckless to hurl myself back into a world of 'normal' people but then again, who is normal?

Two years later, I was delighted when The Priory asked me to arrange DK's retirement party, in June 1999. The obvious venue was the Roehampton Club, where he is a member.

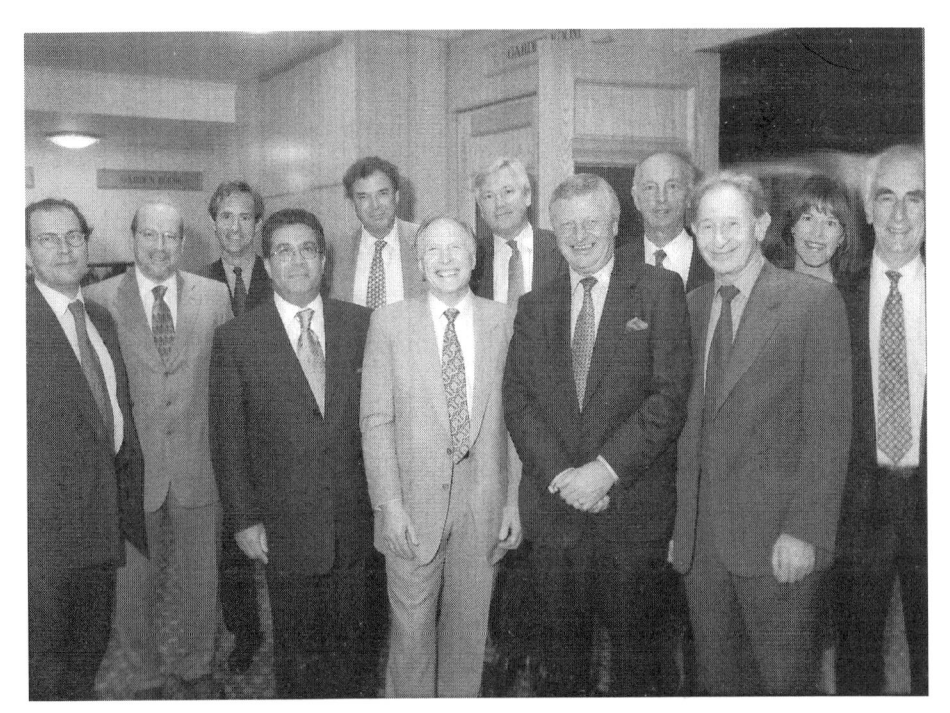

Consultant Psychiatrists at the retirement dinner

From left to right:
Grovelands Priory - Neil Bremer.
Roehampton Priory - Eric Shur, Massimo Riccio, Saeed Islam, Peter Rowan; Desmond Kelly, Mark Collins, David Curson, David Craggs, Dick Penrose; Jeanie Speirs, John Cobb.

During his farewell speech he said:

"...I think of The Roehampton Priory as a catalyst, a test bed of new ideas for private psychiatry in this country. We're out there as pathfinders and our destination will always be excellence. The building – that theatrical Strawberry Hill Gothic extravaganza – appears to have a soul and energy of its own. Put that together with the collective intelligence of a first class staff, and you have something truly unique. As one of the reporters said about The Priory: "I've no idea what it is they've got at this place – but I can see that it definitely works."

Well I'll tell you what it is: we're passionate about our cause, focused in our thoughts, and we care for each other as family. We can only succeed. I'm an extremely lucky fellow to have had the opportunity to be at the helm."

Rory Knight Bruce, in his *Daily Telegraph* article *The man who saved the stars* a few days after the dinner, reported on DK's leaving party:

"While Earnie Larsen, a psychotherapist who had flown in from America to give a speech, pronounced him "a hero whose influence will be felt in 100 years' time", an equally poignant moment came when the tea-lady, Doris Day, who has worked at The Priory for 44 years, made him a presentation. She burst into tears." And John Major sent a message, having sat next to him at an earlier dinner, which summed him up: 'He's nice, he's funny and he's normal.'"

It is surely significant that many staff who became loyal and longstanding employees were anything but keen in their early days. Erich Herrmann handed his notice in within days but stayed 43 years. Had the 'French Sisters' realised that Heathrow was so near, they would have fled, yet Renée chalked up 35 years. Bobby Smith, starting as a kitchen porter in 1980, thought he wouldn't last a week. He is still there.

Together, every one of us helped to rescue the Roehampton Priory from impending bankruptcy and to make it one of the best-known psychiatric hospitals in the country. I was very fortunate to be part of the team.

I could happily continue into my dotage, interviewing people who have worked or stayed at The Priory. Things have changed considerably since the lad James Morgan used to think he would go mad, or be seized, if he ventured within The Priory's forbidding entrance. But there is still much to be done to de-stigmatise psychiatry. I hope that in some small way a look *Inside The Priory* will help.

Just when I thought I was nearing completion of this book, a friend suggested that there should be a thread running through about my own life while working at The Priory. I resisted this idea, feeling that the book should purely be Priory people telling their stories, with me as occasional guide.

But I began to wonder if he didn't have a point? Would it not be an illustration of how so many of us only reveal part of ourselves, the socially acceptable part that seems to glide along relatively smoothly on the surface? Is this not the very essence of the issues addressed at The Priory?

If I was going to write about it, I would need my son's blessing. During an early morning phone call, I asked, "Would you mind if I told our story?" His reaction could not have been more positive: 'I would love to be part of your book' he said, 'include anything you like.'

A few months later, on Friday 20th January 2012, my husband and I were woken by the doorbell at quarter past midnight. Coming out of a deep sleep, I stuck my head out of the window to see who needed us so urgently. Three police officers looked up and said they'd like to come in. We hurried downstairs and Mel ushered them into the kitchen for some reason. As we faced each other, uniforms to dressing gowns, I thought *this won't be good news – should I make tea* – and over their shoulders I was embarrassed to see our cereal bowls set out for the morning, part of Mel's nightly ritual.

One of the officers asked if either of us had a relation living in Bournemouth? "I do, my son," I replied. Could I tell them his name, his date of birth? Then: "I'm sorry to say that your son has passed away. There were no suspicious circumstances, he died peacefully."

As they went on to describe how Rob's flatmate had found him, three hours ago, sitting on the sofa seemingly asleep, his glasses on, a cigarette held in his fingers, I struggled to comprehend their words. Mel must have coaxed me into a chair because suddenly I was standing up again. "No, I think there's been a mistake," I parried, foolishly hopeful. The officers, doubtless used to this sort of denial, stressed that they verified these things very carefully indeed.

When they had gone and we sat together in a daze, I kept thinking *why now?* At a time when he had so much going for him? He was doing well at his job, he was in the third year of his counselling studies, he'd found a counsellor he really liked – why die now?

A week later, seeking solace, we went to see Rob at the Coroner's office, meeting up beforehand with his girlfriend Anne. We sat in a small room while Mike, the Coroner's Officer talked about the (as yet incomplete) post-mortem. A mixture of alcohol and non-dependent drugs had been found in Rob's system but there were further tests to be done. His flatmate had told us that this was Rob's final fling before starting on the course of Librium, which would help him come off alcohol and which waited in the bathroom cabinet.

"Now, are you ready to see Rob?" Mike asked kindly. His choice of words took me back 21 years to the reunion with my son, when the social worker had said, "Are you ready to see him...?" That occasion so full of joy, a new beginning; this one an ending, all hope gone.

I had visualised Mike taking us along dingy corridors to see Rob but he merely took three steps to the opposite wall. "Rob is right here", he said, and at the touch of a button the opaque glass cleared and there was my son, covered in deep blue velvet.

Poor Anne burst into tears and while Mel comforted her, I walked into the room and gazed at this peaceful looking man, my boy. Futile questions and remonstrations teemed through my head but they were no match for my gratitude. *Thank you*, I silently conveyed, *thank you for coming back into my life and making me whole again.*

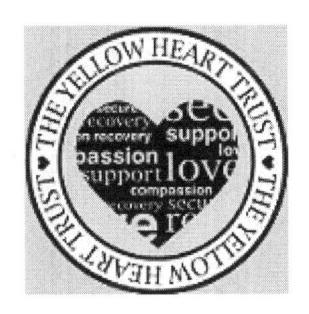

Proceeds of this book go to the Yellow Heart Trust (founded by Alex Fontaine MBE).

The Trust offers compassionate and constructive support for those suffering from unresolved trauma, depression, addiction, dependency and mental health problems.

The Trust recognises that people leaving primary treatment need ongoing help in dealing with all associated problems.

They provide support to men and women with financial restrictions, who need further therapeutic help and assistance towards a more beneficial and fulfilling recovery following initial treatment in whatever form.

For further information see www.yellowheart.org.uk

Registered Charity No: 1093454

Sources

Barr, Ann & York, Peter *The Official Sloane Rangers Handbook.* Ebury Press 1982

Bauml Duberman, Martin *Paul Robeson.* The Bodley Head 1989

Bradford, Sarah *Diana.* Viking 2006

Clapton, Eric, with Simon Sykes, Christopher *Eric Clapton The Autobiography.* Century 2007

Collins, Laura *Kate Moss - the Complete Picture.* Sidgwick & Jackson 2008

Crace, John *The Second Half: thoughts from a male mid-life crisis.* Vista 1998

Durrell, Gerald *Fillets of Plaice.* Collins 1971

Farnes, Norma *Spike an intimate memoir.* Fourth Estate 2003

Gascoigne, Paul with Davies, Hunter *Gazza My Story.* Headline 2004

Howe, David, Sawbridge, Phillida & Hinings, Diana *Half a Million Women.* Penguin Books 1992

Kelly, Desmond *Anxiety and Emotions - physiological basis and treatment.* Charles C Thomas 1980

Larsen, Earnie and Hegarty, Carol *Believing in Myself: Daily Meditations for Healing and Building Self-Esteem.* Simon & Schuster 1991

Larsen, Earnie with Larsen Hegarty, Carol *Now That You're Sober.* Hazelden 2010

Lucas Ogdon, Brenda & Kerr, Michael *Virtuoso: The Story of John Ogdon.* Hamish Hamilton 1981

Pagett, Nicola and Swannell, Graham *Diamonds Behind My Eyes.* Victor Gollancz 1997

Sargant, William *The Unquiet Mind.* William Heinemann Ltd 1967 (2nd edition Pan Books Ltd 1971; reprinted for private distribution 1984 for psychiatric colleagues)

Shorter, Edward *A History of Psychiatry.* John Wiley & Sons, Inc. 1997

Thomas, Jeremy & Hughes, Tony *You Don't Have To Be Famous To Have Manic Depression.* Michael Joseph 2006

Wax, Ruby *How do you want me?* Ebury Press 2002

For the real enthusiast, some seminar examples:

The Treatment of Depression
Thursday 28th January 1982

Introduction: Dr John Horder, President, The Royal College of General Practitioners
The New Antidepressant Drugs
Dr David Wheatley, Twickenham
The Management of Side-Effects and Tricyclic Interactions
Dr George Beaumont, Stockport
Lithium Carbonate Prophylactic Treatment
Dr Alec Coppen, Director MRC Neuropsychiatry Research Laboratory, Epsom
Overcoming Depression
Dr Desmond Kelly, Medical Director, The Priory Hospital
Discussion: Chairman, Dr John Horder. Opened by Prof. Sir Desmond Pond, Immediate Past President of the Royal College of Psychiatrists

Stress in the Professions
Thursday 10th June 1982

Introduction: Prof. Sir Desmond Pond, Chief Scientist to the DHSS and Immediate Past President of the Royal College of Psychiatrists
Stress and the Heart
Dr Peter Nixon, Consultant Cardiologist, Charing Cross Hospital
Starting a New Television Channel – an Exercise in Stress?
Mr Frank McGettigan, Head of Administration, Channel 4
Circadian Rhythm Dysfunction and Sleep Disturbance
Group Capt. Anthony Nicholson, RAF Institute of Aviation Medicine, Farnborough
How to Cope with Stress
Dr Desmond Kelly, Medical Director, The Priory Hospital
Relaxation Techniques
Jane Madders, Physiotherapist
Discussion: Chairman, Prof. Sir Desmond Pond

The Treatment of Anxiety
Thursday 23rd June 1983

Introduction: Sir Desmond Pond, Chief Scientist to the DHSS
The Diagnosis of Anxiety
Professor Anthony Clare, St Bartholomew's Hospital
Are Tranquillisers Harmful?
Dr Desmond Kelly, Medical Director, The Priory Hospital
Stress Control for Professionals
Dr Robert Sharpe, The Institute of Behaviour Therapy
The Management of Anxiety in General Practice

Dr David Wheatley, GP, Twickenham

Conundrums in Psychiatry
Thursday 27th October 1983

Chairman's Introduction: Professor Steven Hirsch, Department of Psychiatry, Charing Cross Hospital
The Uselessness of Psychiatric Diagnosis in General Practice
Professor David Goldberg, Department of Psychiatry, University of Manchester
Action in Crisis
Dr Richard Fox, Honorary Consultant Psychiatrist to The Samaritans
First & Second Generation Antidepressants
Dr Desmond Kelly, Medical Director, The Priory Hospital
Treatment of Bulimia Nervosa
Dr Hubert Lacey, Senior Lecturer in Psychiatry, St George's Hospital, SW17

A Psychosomatic Seminar
Thursday 31st May 1984

Introduction: Dr Desmond Kelly, The Priory Hospital
Fits, Faints and Funny Turns
Sir Desmond Pond, Chief Scientist to the DHSS
The Management of Anorexia & Bulimia Nervosa
Professor Gerald Russell, Institute of Psychiatry and The Maudsley Hospital
New Nutritional Treatment for the Premenstrual Syndrome
Dr Michael Brush, St Thomas's Hospital
Psychosomatic Symptoms and Sex
Dr Patricia Gillan, The Maudsley Hospital

A Stitch in Time
Thursday 11th October 1984

Introduction by the Chairman: Sir Desmond Pond, Chief Scientist to the DHSS
Adolescent Crisis – 'A stitch in time'
Dr Philip Boyd, Consultant Adviser, The Priory Lodge Adolescent Unit
Mind and Myocardial Infarction
Dr Joe Connolly, The Maudsley Hospital
How to Drink Sensibly
Joe Ruzek, Drinkwatchers Study Centre
Professional Burnout and How to Prevent it
Dr Desmond Kelly, The Priory Hospital

Toxic Topics
Thursday 23rd May 1985

Introduction by the Chairman: Professor Ian Brockington, Department of Psychiatry, University of Birmingham

The Toxic Effects of Language upon Medicine
Dr Michael O'Donnell, Author & Broadcaster
The Toxic Effects of Anxiety
Dr John Cobb, Consultant Psychiatrist, The Priory Hospital
The Toxic Effects of Training
Professor Ian Brockington

The William Sargant Lectures
Thursday 3rd October 1985

Introduction by the Chairman: Professor David Goldberg, Department of Psychiatry, University of Manchester
The Anatomy of Healing
Dr Desmond Kelly, Medical Director, The Priory Hospital
Physical Treatment as an Indication of Concern for the Patient
Dr Jim Birley, Dean, The Royal College of Psychiatrists
Therapeutic Effects of the Medical Encounter
Professor David Goldberg
The Classification and Treatment of Anxiety
Dr Peter Tyrer, Consultant Psychiatrist, Mapperley Hospital
Sexual Dysfunction – Organic or Psychiatric?
Dr Peter Gautier-Smith, Consultant Physician, The National Hospital, Queen Square

Update Seminar
Thursday 1st May 1986

Introduction by the Chairman: Sir Desmond Pond, Past President of The Royal College of Psychiatrists
A.I.D.S. – The Present Position
Dr A J Pinching, Senior Lecturer in Immunology, St Mary's Hospital Medical School
Prodromal Schizophrenia – Implications for Outpatients
Professor Steven Hirsch, Charing Cross Hospital Medical School
Communication in Medicine
Dr Michael Smith, Journalist and Broadcaster
Brain Scans – Recent Developments
Dr John Meadows, Consultant Neurologist, Parkside Hospital
Behaviour Therapy – An Update
Dr John Cobb, The Priory Hospital

Winning The Battle
Thursday 25th September 1986

A Tribute to Sir Desmond Pond, Past President of The Royal College of Psychiatrists
Dr Desmond Kelly

Seasonal Affective Disorder and Phototherapy
Dr Christopher Thompson, Senior Lecturer, Charing Cross Hospital
Acute Combat Stress Reactions
Brigadier (Retired) P.D. Wickenden, Emeritus Professor of
Military Psychiatry
Defeating Alcoholism – The Minnesota Model
Dr Desmond Kelly, Medical Director, The Priory Hospital
Stopping Smoking: Where There's a Will
Gillian Riley, Full Stop Programme, Hospital of St John & St Elizabeth

The Sir Desmond Pond Lectures
Thursday 7th May 1987

A Tribute to Sir Desmond Pond, Past President of The Royal College of Psychiatrists
Professor Michael Gelder, University Department of Psychiatry, Oxford
Panic Attacks and Anxiety: New Approaches to an Old Problem
Professor Michael Gelder
The Treatment of Schizophrenia
Professor John Cooper, Department of Psychiatry, Nottingham
Ethical Problems in the Psychiatry of Old Age
Professor Brice Pitt, St Mary's Hospital Medical School, London
Current Issues in Mental Health Legislation
Professor Robert Bluglass, Department of Psychiatry, Birmingham

Cognitive Therapy in Clinical Practice
Thursday 4th May 1989

Chairman: Dr John Cobb, Consultant Psychiatrist, The Priory Hospital
A Cognitive Behavioural Approach to Hypochondriasis
Dr Hilary Warwick, Research Fellow, University Department of Psychiatry, Warneford Hospital, Oxford
Cognitive Therapy in the Management of Breast Cancer
Dr Stirling Moorey, Hon. Senior Registrar, Psychological Medicine, Royal Marsden Hospital
Cognitive Therapy for Survivors of Disasters
Dr Ruth Williams, Lecturer in Psychology, Institute of Psychiatry

Crisis and Consequence
Thursday 5th October 1989

Chairman: Dr Desmond Kelly, Medical Director, The Priory Hospital
Acute Stress Reactions
Dr John Cobb, Clinical Tutor, The Priory Hospital
Suicide and Psychiatric Emergencies
Dr Saeed Islam, Director, Emergency Service, The Priory Hospital
Crisis Intervention in Alcohol Dependence

Dr David Craggs, Medical Director, Galsworthy Lodge
Management of Disasters: The Zeebrugge Experience
Dr Peter Storey, Visiting Consultant, The Priory Hospital

Southern Division Meeting of The Royal College of Psychiatrists
Thursday 2nd November 1989

Chairman of the Southern Division, Dr J J Cockburn
The White Paper Proposals – What Next?
Dr J L T Birley, President, The Royal College of Psychiatrists
Closing a Large Mental Hospital – Problems and Opportunities
Professor Julian Leff, Director, MRC Social Psychiatry Unit,
The Institute of Psychiatry
The Future of the Mental Health Act Commission
Mr Louis Blom-Cooper, Q.C., Chairman, Mental Health Act Commission

The Priory Fellows Research Symposium
Thursday 8th February 1990

Chairperson, Morning Session: Professor Rachel Rosser, Head of Department,
University College and Middlesex Hospital School of Medicine (UCMSM)
Introduction: The Priory Fellowship Scheme
Dr John Cobb, Clinical Tutor and Dr Eric Shur, Fellowship Tutor, The Priory Hospital
Quality of Life – The Measurement of Health
Dr Richard Allison, Clinical Lecturer/Senior Registrar, UCMSM
Student Attitudes to Psychiatry and Psychiatric Clerkship
Dr Catherine O'Brien, Senior Registrar, UCMSM
The Characteristics of Familial Schizophrenia
Dr Tim Read, Senior Registrar, UCMSM
The Frontal Lobe in Schizophrenics and their Relatives
Dr Gerard Bagley, Senior Registrar, St James's Hospital, Portsmouth
Brain Mapping Research at The Priory
Dr Peter Fenwick, Director, Neurophysiology Services, The Priory Hospital
Psychiatry in America
Richard Conte, Executive Vice-President, Community Psychiatric Centers

Chairperson, Afternoon Session: Professor Steven Hirsch, Head of Department,
Charing Cross and Westminster Medical School
Ten Years at The Priory: A Comparison of an NHS and an Independent Hospital
Dr Desmond Kelly, Medical Director
Localisation of a Susceptibility Locus for Schizophrenia on Chromosome 5
Dr Mark Potter, Senior Registrar, UCMSM
(Chairpersons: Dr Hugh Gurling, Senior Lecturer, UCMSM and Professor
Valerie Cowie, Visiting Consultant, The Priory Hospital)

Trial of Brief Intermittent Neuroleptic Prophylaxis for Selected Schizophrenic Outpatients
Dr Anthony Jolley, Consultant Psychiatrist, Charing Cross Hospital
Research from The Priory Bulimia Clinic: Menstrual Disorder and Bulimia
Dr Sara McCluskey, Priory Research Fellow, St George's Hospital Medical School
(Chairperson: Dr Hubert Lacey, Reader and Head of Adult Psychiatry Section, St George's Hospital Medical School)
Psychophysiological Mechanisms of Symptom Production in Irritable Bowel Syndrome (IBS)
Dr Sue Catnach, Priory Fellow, Department of Gastroenterology, St Bartholomew's Hospital
(Chairpersons: Dr Gerald Libby, Medical Director, The Priory Lister Unit (Level 6) and Dr Michael Farthing, Reader in Gastroenterology, St Bartholomew's Hospital)

INDEX

A Problem Aired 90
Ackner, Dr Brian 159
Alcoholics Anonymous (AA) 128,129, 133,135,136,138,139,142,143,177, 195
Alex 141-146
All Saints' Hospital 95
Allison, Dr Richard 37
Altrincham Priory 77
An Introduction to Physical Methods of Treatment 115
Ann 132
Anne 208
Appadoo, Danny 60
Atkinson Morley's Hospital (AMH) 5, 6, 27, 157,166
Aziz 76

Ball, Christina (Chris) 57,133,139-141,143,146,148,151,183
Ballard, Dr Margaret 106-108
Banstead Hospital 159
Barnes Herald 50
Basle University 33
Battle for the Mind 115,117
Baudonne, Renée 22-26, 28, 76, 88, 206
Baudonne, Camille 22-26, 28, 76, 88
Bauml Duberman, Martin 159
Believing in Myself 185
Belmont Hospital 115, 120
Bernard, Sir Thomas x
Berra, Yogi 39
Bethlem Royal Hospital (Bedlam) x, 160
Bewley, Dr Thomas 33
Bob 86, 109, 110,111,124
Bowden House Clinic 11,164
British Journal of Psychiatry 118,120
Brown, Dr Basil 50, 51, 52
Burchill, Julie 148
Burton, Dr Ralph 193-195

Caldicott, Dr Fiona 187,198
Campbell, Alastair 163
Capio Nightingale Hospital 35,36
Charing Cross Hospital 34, 36, 38, 42, 44, 102
Charter Clinic, Chelsea 100
Charter Medical 12, 14, 80
Clapton, Eric 57, 59, 141, 146,147, 184

Clarke, Kenneth 194
Cobb, Dr John 36, 87-92, 100, 169, 170, 171, 205
Collins, Joan 57
Collins, Laura 148
Collins, Dr Mark 99-104, 105, 109, 142, 143, 144, 145, 172, 173,174, 204, 205
Committee for Alcoholics and Vagrants 128
Community Psychiatric Centers (CPC) 11, 63, 73, 74, 76, 77, 123, 157
Conte, Jim 76
Conte, Richard 76, 81
Coppen, Dr Alec 36
Cosmopolitan 176
Coulsdon Hospital 131
Coyle, Peter 70, 129-131, 135
Coyle, Sheila 45, 53, 70, 71, 130, 175
Crace, John 171
Craggs, Dr David 40, 43, 102, 148, 205
Craig, Sir James Henry x
Crisp, Professor Arthur 95, 100, 190
Cruise, Tom 57
Cutting Edge: Against My Nature 168
Cygnet Health Care 11

Dad 81,82,83, 84
Daily Express xi, 162
Daily Mail 30, 176
Daily Telegraph 206
Dally, Dr Peter 95
Davies, Dr Glyn 31, 72, 108
Day, Doris 16, 49, 54-56, 58, 76, 159, 206
Defeat Depression Campaign 189,193
Dempster, Nigel, 30
Depression Alliance 103
Depp, Johnny 148
Derenthal, Bob 74
Dermot 135-138
Diamonds Behind My Eyes 163
Dob, Pene 148, 179-180
Dorchester Hotel 57
Driscoll, Margarette 199
Durack, Ida 25
Durrell, Gerald 23, 25

Eating Disorders Unit (EDU) 42,136, 179,190,204

219

English Nursing Board 21, 34

Falloon, Dr Ian 36
Farnes, Norma 161
Father Tom 130
Fenwick, Dr Peter 197
Fillets of Plaice, 25
Fitznells Manor General Practice 193-195
Flamm, Professor Gerald 2,3,4,8
Flood, Dr John, 5, 6,12,13, 22, 24, 26, 27, 54, 62, 63, 64, 88, 106,121,122 123,133,157,159
Forsyth, Dr Thomas 50, 51, 201, 202
Foundling Hospital x
Frances 155
Franks, Alan 148, 149
Freud, Professor Dr Sigmund 2,163

Galsworthy House (Kingston Hill) 12, 33, 70, 127, 128, 129, 130, 131, 132, 133,134,135,136,137,139,140,180
Galsworthy, John 127
Galsworthy Lodge (in Priory grounds) 41, 57, 101, 102, 127, 148
Garden Wing (ward) 25, 164
Gascoigne, Paul (Gazza) 57, 59, 147, 148
Gelder, Professor Michael 157
Gill, Nicola 176
Glatt, Dr Max 128-129, 130, 132, 137, 150
Goldberg, Professor Sir David 118
Gough, A D vi, x
Graves, Robert 115
Gray, Laura (Bobbie) 49-51
Gready, Bridie 13, 122
Greater London Council 6
Grovelands Priory 116, 187, 188
GROW 195
Guagueta, Clara 56-58, 143, 191
Guy's Hospital 131
Gwatkin, Peter 63

Hanwell Mental Hospital 114
Harley Street, 29, 106
Hauser, Dr Renate 33
Hayes Grove Priory 53, 73
Hegarty, Carol 185
HRH the Princess of Wales 187-191
Herrmann, Erich 26, 51-54, 55, 59, 60, 61, 62, 63, 76, 136, 137, 201, 206
Herrmann, Joyce 158, 201

Hill, Sir Austin Bradford 118
Hopkins, Gerard Manley 39
HSBC 81
Hughes, John, 11-17, 27, 33, 53, 60, 70, 73, 74, 75, 77, 116, 123, 129, 133, 136, 140, 158
Hughes, Dr Tony 185
Hume, Cardinal Basil 30
Hungerford, Mr John 181
Huxley, Aldous 115

International Stress Management Association (ISMA) 196-197
Ironside, Virginia 172
Islam, Dr Saeed 25, 33, 36, 37, 92, 96, 122, 179, 205

James, Harry 52, 54
Jenkins, Dr Rachel 187
Jervis, Virginia 43, 69-70, 89, 155, 203
Johnson, Rev'd Malcolm 131

Kelly, Dr Desmond x, 5-7, 8, 9, 17, 18, 22, 24, 25, 26, 29, 33, 34, 35, 40, 42, 45, 46, 53, 57, 69, 70, 72, 73, 74, 87, 92, 95, 100, 101, 102, 103, 106, 109, 113, 115, 117, 118, 121, 123, 129, 133, 136, 138, 139, 140, 153, 155, 158, 161, 162, 163, 164, 165, 166, 168, 169, 176, 179, 183, 184, 185, 187, 190, 193, 194, 195, 196, 197, 198, 199, 205, 206
Kelly, Marianne 153
Kendrick, Lesley 104-106, 143
Kenneth 132
Kensington House xii
Keogh, Father Cornelius (Con) 195
Kidman, Nicole 57
Kielholz, Professor 164
Kilshaw, Jean 187, 197
King Edward Memorial Hospital 180
King-Lewis, Dr Peter 204
King's Institute of Psychiatry 175
Kingston Hospital 21, 34
Knight Bruce, Lady Eliza x
Knight Bruce, Sir James Lewis x, xi
Knight Bruce, Rory xi, 206

Lacey, Professor Hubert 190
Larsen, Earnie 183-186, 206
Larsen, Paula 183, 184, 185
Led Zeppelin 47
Lewis, Professor Sir Aubrey 90, 118,

Index

Libby, Dr Gerald 37
Lincoln Williams, Dr Edward 131
Logie, Elizabeth 100
London Lighthouse 81
Long, Dr Rodney 131-132, 133
Long Grove Hospital 21, 34
Lower Court (ward) 76, 121
Lower South (ward), 26
Lucas, Brenda 160, 161

MacAuley, Sister Eileen 14, 16, 119-121, 122
Macdonald Wallace, Joe 196
Mackay, Dianne 153-155, 203
Maharishi Mahesh Yogi 7
Major, John 206
Mapother, Professor Edward 115
Marchwood Priory 60, 61
Marianne 169-171
Marie Claire 27
Marie Therese, 27
Marks, Professor Isaac 90
Marsh, Mr Henry, 23, 168
Marsh, Mr John 62
Maudsley Hospital 36, 87, 89, 90, 95, 97, 100, 115, 118, 197
Max Glatt Unit 150
McCluskey, Dr Sara 198
McPhillips, Dr Mike 26, 35, 40-43
Medical Research Council 90
Mel 150, 177, 207, 208
Mercury Development Capital (Mercury Asset Management in 1996) 73, 81
Merton, Sutton & Wandsworth Area Health Authority 21
Metanoia Trust 199
Michael 164-166
Milligan, Spike 161
Mitchell, Laura 196
Moran, Lord Charles Wilson 114
Morgan, James x, 206
Moses 64
Mum 4, 82-86, 109, 167
Murphy, Glorianna, 26-29, 56
Murphy, Rita 132-135, 140

Narcosis 16, 113, 119, 120, 122, 123, 161
Narcosis Unit/Ward 15, 16, 87, 113, 117, 119,
National Health Service (NHS), 5, 6, 12, 21, 33, 35, 36, 40, 41, 42, 43, 44, 73, 75, 76, 77, 79, 80, 87, 88, 95, 96, 97, 100, 101, 102, 105, 113, 128, 142, 153, 162, 190, 194, 197
Naudeer, Betty, 21, 27, 69, 88
Neville-Smith, Graeme 132-135
New Wing (ward), 26, 28
North Wing (ward) 15
Now That You're Sober 186
Nursing Focus 21, 193

Obama, President Barack 118
Ogdon, John 160-161
Outlook 130
Owen, David 117
Owen, Judith 174
Oxford Health Authority 197

Pagett, Nicola 163-164
Patrick 191
Peake, Maeve 159
Peake, Mervyn 159-160
Pedro 202
Pepe 59
Pierre et Marie Curie University 197
Pile, Stephen 196
Pink Floyd 47, 72
Post-Adoption Centre 124
Prestwood, Chris 204
Private One 2, 3
Priory Hospitals Group (PHG) 40, 187, 197, 198
Priory Hospitals Group News 197, 198
Priory Lodge 12, 59, 127, 133,141 [renamed Galsworthy Lodge]
Priory Research Fellowship 42, 190
Purves, Libby 187
Putney Samaritans 198-199

Queen Mary's Hospital 21, 26, 62

Regents Park Nursing Home 132
Reynolds, Ian 81
Richmond Park 37, 46, 63, 91, 127, 135, 144, 165, 181, 185
Ritz, the 57, 143
Robert/Rob 18, 19, 45, 46, 65, 66, 71, 72, 82, 86, 109, 110, 111, 124, 149, 150, 151, 177, 178, 207, 208
Robeson, Ellie 159
Robeson, Paul 159
Robinson, Philip 145
Robson, Bryan 147, 148
Roehampton Club 181, 205
Rosser, Professor Rachel 39, 40

Roumieu, R L vi, x
Rowan, Dr Peter 190, 191, 205
Rowlands, Dr Michael 33
Royal College of General Practitioners 34, 193
Royal College of Physicians 99, 100, 198
Royal Colllege of Psychiatrists 33, 36, 43, 98, 117, 187, 189, 193, 198
Royal College of Surgeons 118
Royal Free and University College Medical School (RFUCMS) ix, 44
Royal Society of Medicine 24, 184
Russell, Bertrand 115
Russell, Professor Gerald 95
Russian Consulate 35

St Augustine's Hospital 187
St Bartholomew's Hospital 99
St Bernard's Hospital 114, 140
St George's Hospital 5, 6, 21, 34, 42, 44, 77, 87, 88, 89, 100, 102, 114, 190
St Raphael's Hospital 1
St Thomas' Hospital 113, 118, 120
Sargant, Dr William 36, 54, 87, 113-119, 122, 123
Sargant, Mrs Peggy 117
Scott, Dr Allan, 24
Settelen, Peter 188
Shanahan, Dr Bill 35-39, 42
Shapiro, Dr Francine 103
Shulman, Senator Joe, 2
Shur, Dr Eric 88, 92, 94, 95-99, 204, 205
Sicks, Dr Timothy 33
Slater, Dr Eliot 115
Smith, Robert (Bobby) 59-60, 143, 206
Smith, Mr 56
Soviet Institute of Psychiatry 35
Speirs, Dr Jeanie 40, 43, 92-95, 205
Spike, An Intimate Memoir 161
Springfield Hospital 88
Spry, Ernest 198
Stage II Recovery: Life Beyond Addiction 185
Steele, Richard 139, 141
Steve the Falconer 31
Stoppard, Dr Miriam 187
Storey, Dr Peter 36, 100
Suter, Brian 52, 60-64, 117, 135, 137
Sutton Emergency Hospital 115
Sutton General Hospital, 33

Swindlehurst, Rob 100

Ted the Herdsman 50, 51
Terrence Higgins Trust 81
Thames Television 90, 91
Thatcher, Margaret 39, 91
The British Medical Journal 34
The Mind Possessed 117
The Mirror 52, 105, 149
The Official Sloane Ranger Handbook ix
The Primal Scream 109
The Second Half: thoughts from a male mid-life crisis 172
The Sunday Times 196, 199
The Unquiet Mind 115, 117
Thomas, Jeremy 185, 186
Thompson, Dr David 17, 36
Thomson, Dr Morven 25, 33, 122-124
Tony (cook) 16
Tony (nurse) 143
Transcendental Meditation (TM) 7, 103
Treatment Corridor (ward) 26, 27, 28, 50
Trimble, Dr Michael 168
TTP Counselling Centre 151
Turning Point charity 187, 189
Tyrer, Dr Peter 118

University College and Middlesex School of Medicine (UCMSM) 39
University of Edinburgh 196
University of Oxford 36
University of Sussex 196
Upper Court (ward) 60, 170
Upper South (ward) 26
Upper West (ward) 28
Upstairs Downstairs 163

Vinacour, Mr 63

Wakefield, David 73-81, 87
Wallace, Rose 45, 46, 65, 66
Warlingham Park Hospital 128
Watney, John 159
Watts, Florence 54
Wax, Ruby ix, 103, 172-175, 180
Wells, Dr Brian 38
West Wing (ward), 23
Westminster Advisory Centre on Alcoholism 132
Westminster Counselling Service 139
Westminster Healthcare 80
Westminster Hospital 92

Whear, John 60-64
White, Adrian, Carolyn, Christine, Helen and Ruth 71
White, Jim 71, 82, 84, 85
White, Susan 35, 72, 82, 85, 196
Woman's Hour 189
Wood, Dr William ix, xi, xii, 5, 137, 201
Wood Wing (ward) 60
Woodbourne Clinic 73

Yeats, W.B. 39
Yellow Heart Trust 145, 146, 209
You Don't Have to be Famous to Have Manic Depression 185

Zander, Benjamin 82